A CHINESE MEDICINE GEOMETRICAL HEALING HANDBOOK

Denys & Victor Jacques

Discovery Publisher

©2020, Discovery Publisher
All rights reserved

No part of this book may be reproduced in any form or by any electronic or mechanical means including information storage and retrieval systems, without permission in writing from the publisher.

Authored by Denys and Victor Jacques
Translated by Michel Bosc and Julien Bringuier

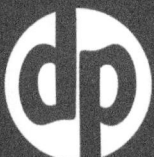

616 Corporate Way
Valley Cottage, New York
www.discoverypublisher.com
editors@discoverypublisher.com
Proudly not on Facebook or Twitter

New York • Paris • Dublin • Tokyo • Hong Kong

TABLE OF CONTENTS

A CHINESE MEDICINE GEOMETRICAL HEALING HANDBOOK — 1
DENYS & VICTOR JACQUES — 1

FOREWORD — 2

I – THE ENERGETIC PALPATION — 4
A – INTERROGATING THE BODY TISSUES AS A TOOL FOR RESEARCH — 4
B – INFORMATION AS A CORRECTION TOOL — 7

II – ANATOMICAL DECODING — 9
A – HAND DECODING — 9
I – HORIZONTAL INTERROGATION ON THE SURFACE (EPIDERMIS) — 9
II – VERTICAL INTERROGATION AT THE OSSEOUS LEVEL — 10
III – HORIZONTAL INTERROGATION AT THE OSSEOUS LEVEL — 11
B – MUSCLE DECODING — 15

III – ENERGY MOVEMENT OF THE VISCERA — 27

IV – THE PHASES OF DISEASE — 30
PHASE I: ELIMINATION — 30
PHASE II: INFLAMMATION (REACTION) — 30
PHASE III: DEPOSITION — 30
PHASE IV: IMPREGNATION — 31
PHASES V: DEGENERATION — 31
PHASE VI: NEOPLASM — 32

THE READING GRID — 35
V – INTRODUCTION TO THE READING GRID — 36

THE CENTRES   41

VI – INTRODUCTION TO THE CENTRES   42

I – PALPATION OF THE CENTRE   42

II – DETERMINING THE DISTURBED EXTRAORDINARY CHANNEL OR CHAIN   42

III – DETERMINING THE DISTURBED ENERGETIC FUNCTION ON THE CHAIN OR EXTRAORDINARY CHANNEL   42

IV – CORRECTION   43

VII – FRONT-MU POINTS AND BACK-SHU POINTS   46

I – OVERALL CONTROL OF THE 3 LEVELS   47

II – DETERMINING THE DISTURBED LEVEL (S)   48

III – DETERMINING THE DISTURBED ENERGETIC FUNCTION   48

IV – CORRECTION   49

VIII – THE EMOTIONAL CHAINS OF THE DU MAI, STOMACH AND GALL BLADDER CHANNELS   53

A – THE EMOTIONAL CHAIN OF THE DU MAI   53

I – OVERALL CONTROL OF THE DU MAI   54

II – DETERMINING THE DISTURBED VERTEBRAL OR CRANIAL AREA   55

III – DETERMINING THE DISTURBED ENERGETIC FUNCTION (IN RESONANCE BLOCKAGE)   55

IV – CORRECTION   57

B – THE EMOTIONAL CHAIN OF THE STOMACH CHANNEL   57

I – OVERALL CONTROL OF THE STOMACH EMOTIONAL CHAIN   58

II – DETERMINING THE DISTURBED ENERGETIC FUNCTION   58

III – CORRECTION   59

C – THE EMOTIONAL CHAIN OF THE GALL BLADDER CHANNEL   60

I – OVERALL CONTROL   61

II – DETERMINING THE DISTURBED ENERGETIC FUNCTION   61

III – CORRECTION   61

- D – OVERALL CONTROL OF THE 3 EMOTIONAL CHAINS (DU MAI-STOMACH-GALL BLADDER) ON THE METATARSAL DORSAL SIDE ... 63
- E – OVERALL CONTROL: THE VERTEX CENTRE ... 63

IX – THE EXTRAORDINARY CHANNELS ... 64
- A – THERAPEUTIC LEVELS AND CENTRES ... 65
- B – THE CENTRAL EXTRAORDINARY CHANNELS ... 67
  - REN MAI (CENTRAL RESERVOIR OF YIN ENERGIES) ... 67
    - I – OVERALL CONTROL ... 67
    - II – CORRECTION ... 68
  - DU MAI (CENTRAL RESERVOIR OF YANG ENERGIES) ... 69
  - CHONG MAI "THE SEA OF THE 5 ORGANS AND 6 VISCERA" (LING SHU) ... 69
    - I – OVERALL CONTROL ... 69
    - II – DERTERMINING THE DISTURBED ENERGETIC FUNCTION ... 70
    - III – CORRECTION ... 70
  - DAI MAI ... 70
    - I – OVERALL CONTROL ... 70
    - II – CORRECTION ... 70
- C – THE SECONDARY EXTRAORDINARY CHANNELS ... 70
  - I – OVERALL CONTROL ... 71
  - II – CORRECTION ... 71
- D – THE MASTER POINTS ... 72
  - I – OVERALL CONTROL ... 72
  - II – DETERMINING THE AFFECTED MASTER POINT ... 72
  - III – CORRECTION ... 72
- E – THE CEPHALIC PSYCHO-SOMATIC GENERATOR = GB 1 TO GB 9 POINTS ... 72
  - I – OVERALL CONTROL ... 73
  - II – DETERMINING THE AFFECTED EXTRAORDINARY CHANNEL ... 73
  - III – CORRECTION ... 73
- F – MUSCLE DECODING ... 73

X – THE SPECIFIC CENTRE OF THE GALL BLADDER CHANNEL — 76
I – OVERALL CONTROL — 76
II – CORRECTION — 76

XI – THE SPECIFIC CENTRES OF THE SPLEEN — 78
A – CENTRE OF THE SPLEEN CHANNEL (SP 1 TO SP 11) — 78
I – BLOOD PRODUCTION — 78
II – IMMUNE DEFENCE — 78
B – CENTRE OF THE SPLEEN CHAIN — 78
I – SPECIFIC CONTROL — 79
II – DETERMINING THE DISTURBED ENERGETIC FUNCTION — 79
III – CORRECTION — 80

XII – THE SPECIFIC CENTRE OF THE HEART CHANNEL — 82
I – OVERALL CONTROL — 82
II – DETERMINING THE DISTURBED POINT OF THE HEART CHANNEL — 82
III – CORRECTION — 82

XIII – THE OCCIPITAL CENTRE — 84
A – THE OUTER PATHWAY OF THE URINARY BLADDER CHANNEL — 84
I – OVERALL CONTROL — 84
II – DETERMINING THE DISTURBED ENERGETIC FUNCTION — 85
III – CORRECTION — 85
B – UB 31 TO UB 35 POINTS — 85
I – OVERALL CONTROL — 85
II – CORRECTION — 85

XIV – THE FRONTAL CENTRE — 87
I – DETERMINING THE AFFECTED CHANNEL — 87
II – CORRECTION — 87

XV – THE PHYSICAL TRAUMA — 88
A – THE TRAUMATIC BLOCKAGES — 88
- I – OVERALL CONTROL — 88
- II – CORRECTION — 88

B – TENDINITIS — 90
- I – OVERALL CONTROL — 90
- II – CORRECTION — 90

XVI – THE BARRIERS — 92
- I – OVERALL CONTROL — 92
- II – DETERMINING THE AFFECTED ENERGETIC FUNCTION — 92
- III – CORRECTION — 93

COMPLEMENTARY CONTROLS — 95

XVII – THE WINDOW OF THE SKY POINTS — 96
- I – OVERALL CONTROL — 96
- II – CORRECTION — 96

A – THE TRIPLE WARMER — 98
- I – OVERALL CONTROL — 98
- II – CORRECTION — 98

B – THE SP 6 POINT — 99
- I – OVERALL CONTROL — 99
- II – CORRECTION — 99

XIX – STOMACH CHAIN AND ENERGY STAGNATION — 100
- I – OVERALL CONTROL — 100
- II – DETERMINING THE LOCATION OF STAGNATION IN THE 3 BURNERS — 100
- III – CORRECTION — 100

XX – THE PERICARDIUM CHANNEL — 102
- I – OVERALL CONTROL — 102

- II – DETERMINING THE DISTURBED POINT ON THE PERICARDIUM CHANNEL — 102
- III – CORRECTION — 103

XXI – CHAIN FROM KD 22 TO KD 27 — 103
- I – OVERALL CONTROL — 103
- II – DETERMINING THE DISTURBED ENERGETIC FUNCTION — 103
- III – CORRECTION — 104

XXII – GENERAL FUNCTIONS — 105
- I – OVERALL CONTROL — 105
- II – SPECIFIC CONTROLS — 105
- III – DETERMINING THE DISTURBED ENERGETIC FUNCTION — 106
- IV – CORRECTION — 106

XXIII – THE LUO POINTS OF THE 12 CHANNELS — 107
- I – OVERALL CONTROL — 107
- II – DETERMINING THE AFFECTED LUO POINT — 107
- III – CORRECTION — 108

XXIV – CIRCULATION BLOCKAGE IN THE 12 CHANNELS — 109
- I – OVERALL CONTROL — 109
- II – DETERMINING THE AFFECTED CHANNEL — 109
- III – CORRECTION — 109

XXV – THE TENDINO-MUSCULAR CHANNELS (JING JIN) — 110
- I – PALPATORY STUDY — 110
- II – OVERALL CONTROL — 111
- III – CORRECTION — 111

XXVI – ELIMINATION FUNCTION OF ST 36 - ST 37 - ST 39 POINTS — 113
- I – OVERALL CONTROL — 113
- II – CORRECTION — 113

XXVII – THE 3 DAN TIAN — 114
I – OVERALL CONTROL — 114
II – SPECIFIC CONTROL OF THE 3 DAN TIAN — 114
III – CORRECTION — 114

XXVIII – COMMENTS ON THE READING GRID — 116

EPILOGUE — 119

AND ANNEXES — 119

EPILOGUE — 121
ANNEX I: SUMMARIZED PLATES — 122
ANNEX II: BIBLIOGRAPHY — 132
ANNEX III: LIST OF ABBREVIATIONS — 134

ACKNOWLEDGMENTS — 137

TABLE OF PLATES

PLATE 1: HORIZONTAL SURFACE INTERROGATION IN THE LONGITUDINAL AXIS OF THE HAND DORSAL SIDE	12
PLATE 2: VERTICAL OSSEOUS INTERROGATION OF THE HAND DORSAL SIDE	13
PLATE 3: HORIZONTAL OSSEOUS INTERROGATION OF THE HAND DORSAL SIDE	14
PLATE 4: "LV CHANNEL" "PC CHANNEL" MUSCLES	17
PLATE 5: "KD CHANNEL" "HT CHANNEL" MUSCLES	18
PLATE 6: "LI CHANNEL" "SP CHANNEL" MUSCLES	19
PLATE 7: "SI CHANNEL" "LU CHANNEL" "UB CHANNEL" MUSCLES	20
PLATE 8: "GB CHANNEL" "TW CHANNEL" MUSCLES	21
PLATE 9: "ST CHANNEL" MUSCLE	22
PLATE 10: "ELEMENT" MUSCLES (I)	23
PLATE 11: "ELEMENT" MUSCLES (II)	24
PLATE 12: "ELEMENT" MUSCLES (III)	25
PLATE 13: "EXTRAORDINARY CHANNELS" MUSCLES	26
PLATE 14: ENERGY MOVEMENT OF THE VISCERA (I)	29
PLATE 15: ENERGY MOVEMENT OF THE VISCERA (II)	29
PLATE 16: THE CENTRES	44
PLATE 17: THE ENERGETIC FUNCTIONS AT THE ANTERIOR SIDE OF THE WRIST	45
PLATE 18: JING BIE SHU/MU POINTS	51
PLATE 19: JING BIE AND FUNCTION SHU/MU POINTS	52
PLATE 20: EMOTIONAL CHAIN OF THE DU MAI	56
PLATE 21: EMOTIONAL CHAIN OF THE STOMACH CHANNEL	59
PLATE 22: EMOTIONAL CHAIN OF THE GALL BLADDER CHANNEL	62

PLATE 23: THE 3 STAGES OF THE ENERGETIC SYSTEM (ACCORDING TO J. PIALOUX)	66
PLATE 24: THE EXTRAORDINARY CHANNELS ON THE HAND DORSAL SIDE (OSSEOUS)	74
PLATE 25: THE EXTRAORDINARY CHANNELS ON THE PELVIS	75
PLATE 26: THE SPECIFIC CENTRE OF THE GALL BLADDER CHANNEL	77
PLATE 27: THE SPECIFIC CENTRE OF THE GALL BLADDER CHANNEL	81
PLATE 28: SPECIFIC CENTRE OF THE HEART CHANNEL	83
PLATE 29: THE OCCIPITAL CENTRE	86
PLATE 30: THE FRONTAL CENTRE	88
PLATE 31: THE PHYSICAL TRAUMA	91
PLATE 32: LOCATION OF THE ENERGETIC FUNCTIONS AT THE DORSAL SIDE OF THE WRIST	93
PLATE 33: THE WINDOW OF THE SKY POINTS XVIII – THE PATHWAY OF LIQUIDS	97
PLATE 34: STOMACH CHAIN AND ENERGY STAGNATION	101
PLATE 35: THE 3 DAN TIAN	115
PLATE 36: THE CENTRES	123
PLATE 37: THE EXTRAORDINARY CHANNELS ON THE HAND DORSAL SIDE (OSSEOUS)	124
PLATE 38: THE ENERGETIC FUNCTIONS AT THE ANTERIOR SIDE OF THE WRIST (SURFACE)	125
PLATE 39: THE ENERGETIC FUNCTIONS AT THE ANTERIOR SIDE OF THE WRIST (DERMIS)	126
PLATE 40: THE ENERGETIC FUNCTIONS AT THE ANTERIOR SIDE OF THE WRIST (OSSEOUS + TENDON)	127
PLATE 41: SUMMARIZED PLATE (SURFACE)	128
PLATE 42: SUMMARIZED PLATE (DERMIS)	129
PLATE 43: SUMMARIZED PLATE (PALM/SURFACE) (I)	130
PLATE 44: SUMMARIZED PLATE (PALM/SURFACE) (II)	131

A CHINESE MEDICINE GEOMETRICAL HEALING HANDBOOK

Denys & Victor Jacques

FOREWORD

This book is essentially practical, intended for readers trained in Chinese Medicine. It does not provide a basic study of points, channels and other fundamental principles presented in many works.

Diagnosis in Traditional Chinese Medicine is mainly given by questioning the patient, inspecting the tongue, the complexion and the nails, abdominal palpating and radial pulse taking. From these elements, the therapist, whose interpretation is not thoroughly free of his (her) own subjectivity, chooses through reasoning to puncture some points with needles, to warm them up with moxas, to massage them or to use cupping glasses. The energetic system however is so complex that there might be a gap or a distortion between the intellectual approach of the practitioner and the energetic reality of the patient.

The object of this book is not to replace the traditional diagnosis methods and needling techniques but to provide an additional tool to enhance the efficiency of treatments. Our perspective is based on a specific palpation of tissues which allows to determine the energetic functions that are disturbed and on what level (physical, emotional or spiritual.)

"Only the tissues know". The therapist does not choose what is right to do for the patient, actually, the tissues show him where the body is in need. For this, we must find a key to reading (how to palpate) and a reading grid (where to palpate).

Through the energetic techniques widely developed here, the therapist can identify a closed point (a point which does not respond to a stimulation) or a stagnation in channels and organs. Acquiring the sensation of the Energy is essential in order to listen to the patient's body.

The principle of resonance is the basis of the reading grid. The energetic system is reflected in the anatomy, in the physical structures: bones, muscles, dermis...We can take as an example the correspondence between the 5 Elements and the 5 metacarpal bones or between the 14 channels (12 main channels, Ren Mai and Du Mai) and the 14 finger phalanges. Their palpation tells us about the energetic disorders.

The correction method – also applicable to the physical trauma- consists in giving the information which allows the body to correct itself. The practitioner only shows the points related to the disturbed energetic functions and determined by the reading grid. These points, then, "respond" and "communicate" again and a change in the tissues is perceived right away under his hands.

The grid was elaborated after many observations which were checked and double checked. We invite the reader to approach this book with an inquiring mind and the desire to experiment on his own our working hypotheses and the points of view that we expressed. We are open to any constructive dialogue.

The authors mean to emphasize that this work could not have been done without the teachings of Jacques Pialoux, Régis Blin and Jean-Pierre Guiliani and we wish to express all our thankfulness and gratitude.

At last, this book would not have been possible without the presence and support of Véronique.

• • •

The deepest thing in man is the skin.
–Paul Valéry

I – THE ENERGETIC PALPATION

A – INTERROGATING THE BODY TISSUES AS A TOOL FOR RESEARCH

Several palpation methods are possible:

- → **Usual palpation** which allows to assess flexibility, heat, shape, mobility of tissues.
- → **Passive listening** which consists in putting hands down and paying attention without inferring anything from what is going on under one's fingers.
- → At last, **active interrogation** which is our main searching tool, our key to reading the body. Using this method, the therapist studies tissue response to a stimulation, to an energetic push generated in his abdomen from the contraction of abdominal muscles and conveyed to tissues through his hands. The therapist does not use only his fingers to question but his whole body.

Two types of active interrogation:

- → "Vertical" interrogation: the impulse, a pressure with one or several fingers of one hand, is given from surface to depth. The practitioner will evaluate whether there is a tissue response to stimulation or not as he wanted to assess "elasticity". In case of blockage, there is little or no response, no rebound.

I – THE ENERGETIC PALPATION

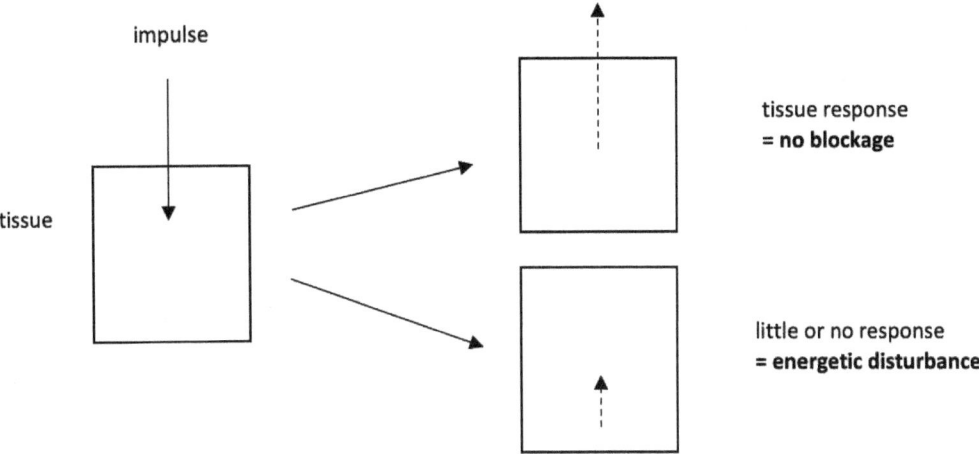

It is important that the impulse be located in the studied tissue (epidermis, dermis, muscle or bone). The practitioner must apply a deep pressure to reach the bone, whereas, to study the epidermis, the stimulation must remain superficial. An acupuncture point will be called "open" if it responds to a vertical impulse on the surface, whether the skin tissue is hard or distended. A point which has lost its Energy does not respond any longer (see drawing below).

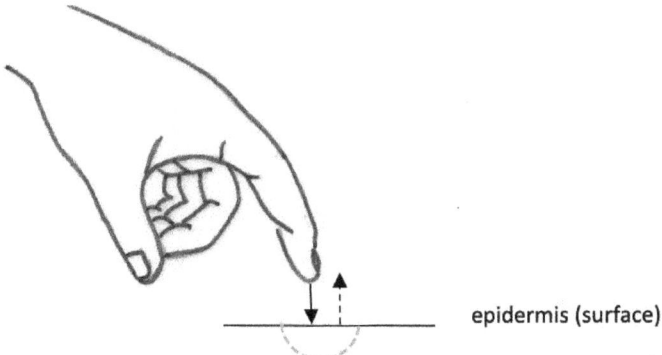

→ "Horizontal" interrogation: the impulse is almost given tangentially to the tissue, in a precise direction.

It induces a minimal movement of the tested tissue which will respond in two possible ways.

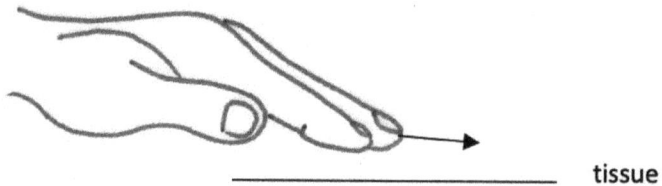

→ Either it is easily penetrated: the therapist does not experience any resistance to his impulse = no blockage.
→ The practitioner feels right away a barrier, a wall that keeps him from going through the tissue = blockage.

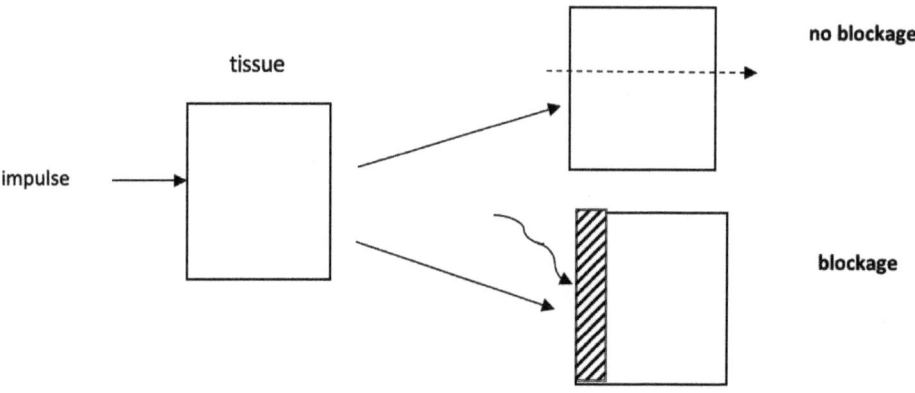

In the reading grid of the body, the impulse is given most often crosswise in relation to the longitudinal axis of the body and the possible blockage only appears in this direction.

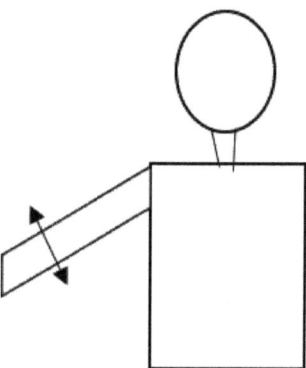

Before interrogating a tissue, the practitioner must be sure he can mobilize it with a usual palpation. If a dermis area is stuck to the underlying layer and if he (she) cannot move it, any interrogation will be impossible on this level (as it can be the case with an acute sprained ankle, serious circulatory disorders or a hand deformed by arthritis). He would find a blockage whatever the direction of the impulse might be. In this case, another area of the body will give the same information with a different palpation.

The interrogation thus made (vertical or horizontal) can cover different structures: a point, a channel, a dermis area, a muscle, an organ, or a bone…).

B – INFORMATION AS A CORRECTION TOOL

If searching is done with one hand, the correction is made with both hands. It consists in connecting the blocked point (related to the disturbed energetic function and determined by the reading grid) to a specific area that will open it. This area may be another point, a channel, an organ, a vertebra…

The therapist, then, feels as if he had a tight "**rope**" between his hands. The sensation is not **under** but **between** the hands and in his abdomen, which is the main receiver of energetic sensations. The practitioner keeps this rope, becomes inactive and waits for the body self-correcting reaction in the next few seconds which translates into the loosening of the rope, both hands do not seem connected anymore. The blocked point responds again and the checking areas that led to its treatment are blockage free.

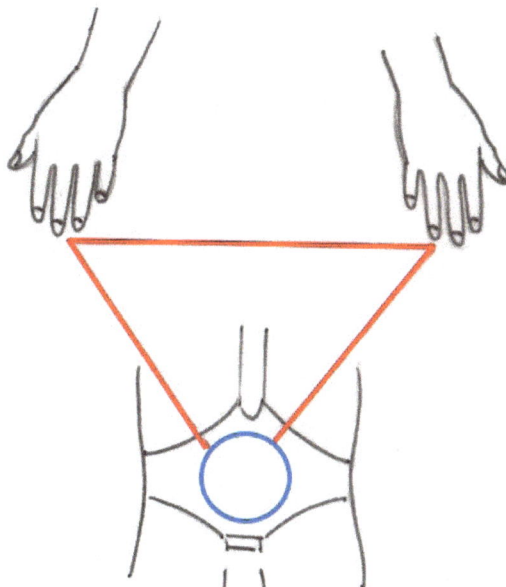

The reading grid that we will study next allows us to know where the body is in need, so we do not push through closed doors - the locked points whose key is to be found elsewhere. It determines the energetic functions that are disturbed and the affected therapeutic levels. The practitioner does not decide what is good for the patient nor bring energy here or there, based upon some intellectual reasoning. He is just giving the information that the patient's body comes to get in order to correct itself - the concept of "no acting" in oriental way of thinking. The practitioner does not have to be concerned about the choice of points, he decides nothing, he only proceeds according to what the tissues tell him.

The palpation technique, as described above, can be learned with some training and practice. However, if one feels with his "guts" - the Hara[1] centre in Japanese philosophy, this area must be free of any tension that might interfere with the received information. A stressed out or anxious therapist with a "knot" in his stomach, or lost in his own thoughts, tired, or disturbed by digestive problems, will not have an accurate perception. The practitioner must be thoroughly available mentally (emptying the mind in some way is essential) as well as physically. This is the main difficulty that we encounter in daily practice. Working on oneself before working on patients is sometimes necessary.

The reading grid confirms, specifies, or invalidates the therapeutic choice considered after the questioning and classic examination. However, reasoning is important, it allows to understand what the practitioner finds out through palpation and to link the patient's symptoms and the reading of the body. Through palpation and reasoning, the therapist has a better understanding of the energetic imbalance.

---
1. Dürckheim Karlfried Graf, *Hara: The Vital Center of Man*, Inner Traditions Publisher

II – ANATOMICAL DECODING

Régis Blin[1] is the author of a remarkable study about the resonance of the energetic system on the anatomic structures.

When an energetic function is disturbed (an Element, a channel…), the physical structures (bones, muscles, viscera…) which are on the same frequency are also disturbed. This chapter refers in part to this study, using the palpation described previously.

The osseous and muscular readings give us information on energetic disorders and their solving in the course of treatment. However, it does not tell us directly which ones need a correction (since a blockage may have different origins) and which therapeutic level (elemental, corporal, emotional, spiritual) is affected. The reading grid will give us this information.

A – HAND DECODING

The study is done according to the palpation mode. One anatomical area can be in relationship and in resonance with different energetic functions depending on the palpation mode that is utilized.

I – HORIZONTAL INTERROGATION ON THE SURFACE (EPIDERMIS)

The index finger of the therapist is laid flat lengthways on the dorsal side of the phalanx or metacarpal bones. The impulse is given horizontally, on the surface.

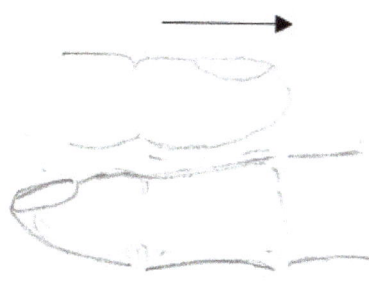

The practitioner's finger may move the patient's epidermis on a very short distance or on the contrary, it may seem to be stuck and cannot be moved in case of a blockage.

---

1. Blin Régis, *L'Hexagramme Tridimensionnel*, S.F.E.R.E.

→ The 12 phalanxes of the 4 fingers (not the thumb) are in resonance with the 12 channels (see plate 1).
→ The 5 metacarpal bones are in resonance with the 5 Elements (see plate 1).

This test on the metacarpal bones gives information mainly about the Yang aspect of each Element, related to the organ or viscera surface, the Back- Shu point, the "5 Element" function, the emotional level…

The phalanx blockage can be confirmed by the palpation of the related channel: the therapist's hand is laid lengthwise on the channel pathway at the leg or forearm level which are easier palpation areas. The practitioner gives a vertical impulse while remaining on the surface. He can evaluate the response or the absence of response of the epidermis in the case of a blockage. It is also possible to test the "channel" muscle related on the lower limb (see muscle decoding in this chapter). To confirm the blockage at the metacarpal level, the practitioner may check the related "Element" muscle on the trunk.

II – VERTICAL INTERROGATION AT THE OSSEOUS LEVEL

The index finger of the therapist is laid flat on the dorsal side of the phalanx or the metacarpal body.

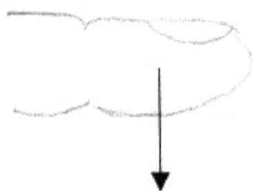

The impulse is vertical from surface to depth towards the osseous level. Is the bone responding as if it were elastic or not in the case of a blockage?

→ The 12 phalanx of the fingers and the 2 of the thumb are in resonance with the 14 bones of the skull and face, which will be also tested with the same palpation, fingers laid flat on the bone itself (for the ones within reach) (see plate 2).
→ The 5 metacarpal bones (except for the head and the base) are in resonance with the 5 Elements (see plate 2).

The test gives information mainly about the Yin of each Element, thus related to the organ or viscera depth, the Mu point, the "3 burner" function of the organ or viscera, the physical level. Confirmation through palpation of the related "Element" muscle on the trunk.

→ The head and base of the 4 last metacarpal bones are in resonance with the Extraordinary Channels at a precise therapeutic level (psychosomatic generator of the head = cephalic control points).

III – HORIZONTAL INTERROGATION AT THE OSSEOUS LEVEL

It concerns the interphalangeal articulations in resonance with the master points of the 8 Extraordinary Channels and the thumb column in resonance with the Extraordinary Channels and their constituent points.

The last phalanx of the therapist's index finger laid flat on the dorsal side of the interphalangeal articulations and of the thumb phalanx and metacarpal bone, laid across the hand longitudinal axis (see plate 3).

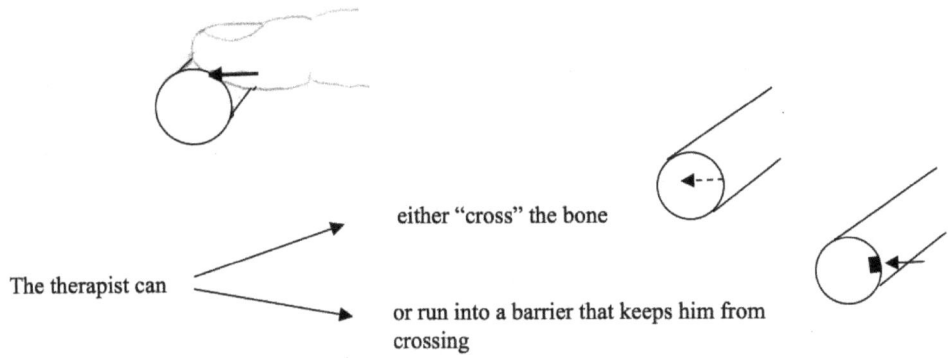

Reminder of master points:

Chong Mai	➡	SP 4
Yin Wei Mai (yWM)	➡	PC 6
Yin Qiao Mai (yQH)	➡	KD 6
Ren Mai (RM)	➡	LU 7
Du Mai (DM)	➡	SI 3
Yang Qiao Mai (YQH)	➡	UB 62
YangWei Mai (YWM)	➡	TW 5
Dai Mai	➡	GB 41

Decoding of the thumb column:

P2	➡	Du Mai

P1 ➡ Ren Mai
M1 head ➡ Chong Mai
M1 neck ➡ Dai Mai
M1 proximal part ➡ Secondary Extraordinary Channels
(see chapter IX on the Extraordinary Channels)

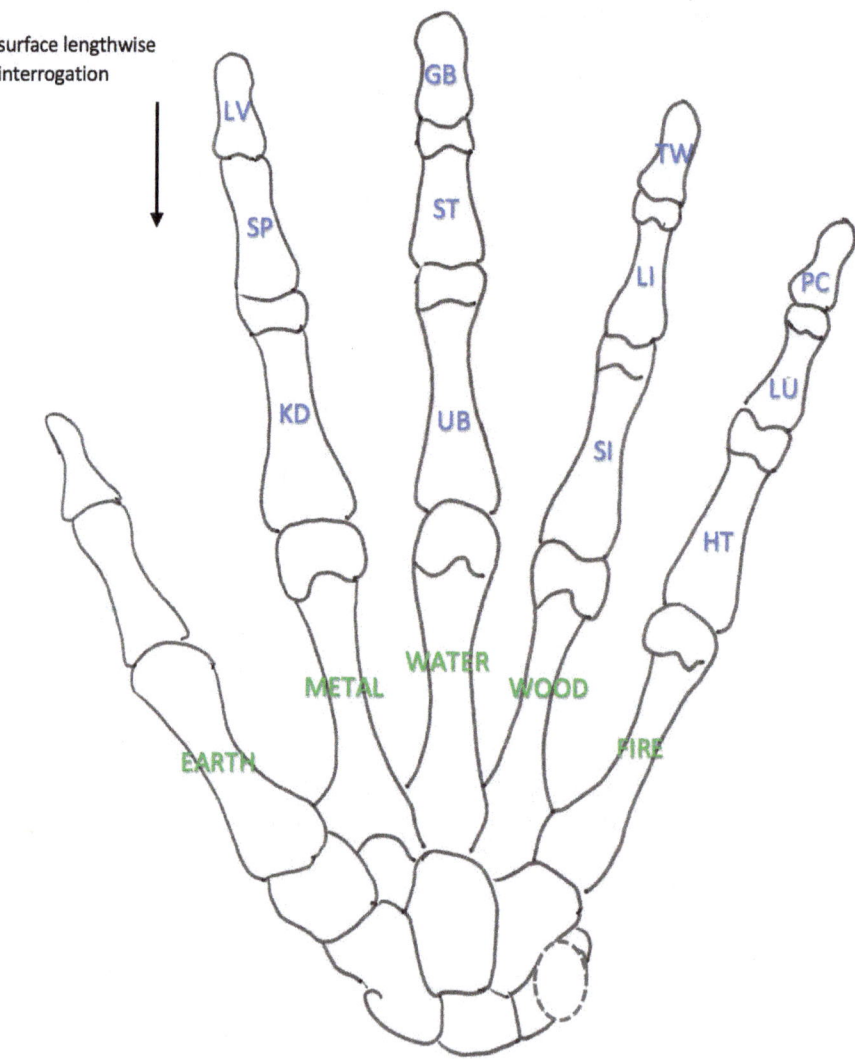

PLATE 1: HORIZONTAL SURFACE INTERROGATION IN THE LONGITUDINAL AXIS OF THE HAND DORSAL SIDE

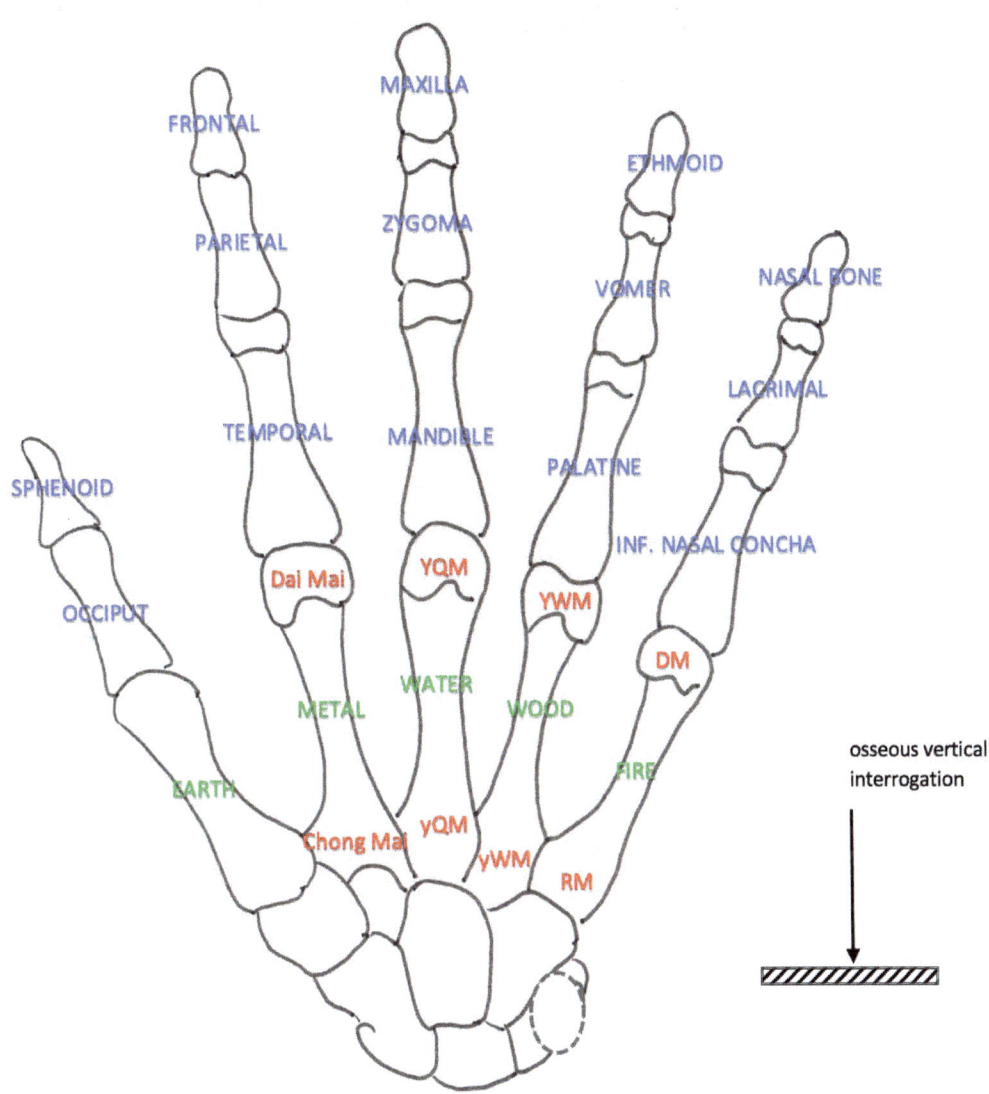

PLATE 2: VERTICAL OSSEOUS INTERROGATION
OF THE HAND DORSAL SIDE

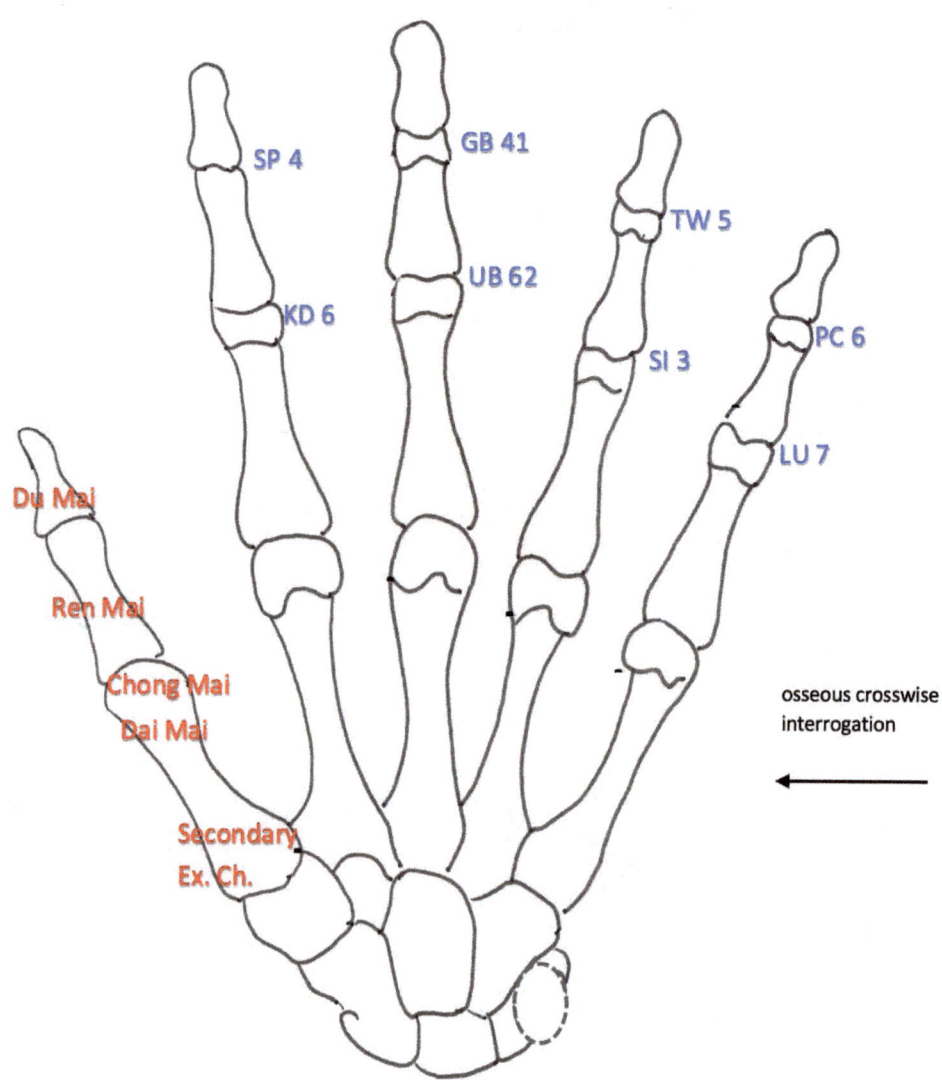

PLATE 3: HORIZONTAL OSSEOUS INTERROGATION OF THE HAND DORSAL SIDE

B – MUSCLE DECODING

→ The muscles in resonance with the 12 channels are tested at the leg and foot level.

→ The muscles in resonance with the 5 Elements are tested at the trunk level, mostly in the lower half.

→ The muscles in resonance with the Extraordinary Channels are the thigh adductors.

The reader will find the complete muscle decoding in the book by Régis Blin.

The interrogation is horizontal with the fingers laid flat at the dermis level (not the epidermis) in the direction of the muscle to test, as described in the following outlines. The therapist may displace the dermis without resistance on a short distance or come up against a barrier right away, his fingers are stopped, the dermis cannot be crossed in case of blockage.

The therapist must make sure the dermis can be mobilized on the underlying tissue with a usual palpation before interrogating it.

	"Channel" muscle	"Element" muscle
LU	→ fibularis tertius m	ilio-costalis m
LI	→ abductor hallucis m	quadratus lumbarum m
	→ abductor digiti minimi m	
SP	→ tibialis posterior m	interspinales m
ST	→ flexor digitorum brevis m	transversus abdominis m
KD	→ flexor hallucis longus m	longissimus m
UB	→ extensor hallucis longus m	rectus abdominis m
HT	→ flexor digitorum longus m	transversospinales m
PC	→ fibularis longus m	latissimus dorsi m
TW	→ soleus + 2 gastrocnemus m	trapezius m
LI	→ fibularis brevis m	serratus posterior superior m
		serratus posterior inferior m
GB	→ tibialis anterior m	external oblique m

In the plates of following pages:

→ The preferential palpation areas and the impulse direction are underlined in blue for the « channel » muscles. The impulse, lengthwise, can be given in both directions (from top to bottom and from bottom to top).

→ La The palpation areas and the impulse direction are indicated with arrows for the « Element » muscles.

Note:

→ This reading does not concern muscular trauma that will be studied in chapter XV.

II – ANATOMICAL DECODING

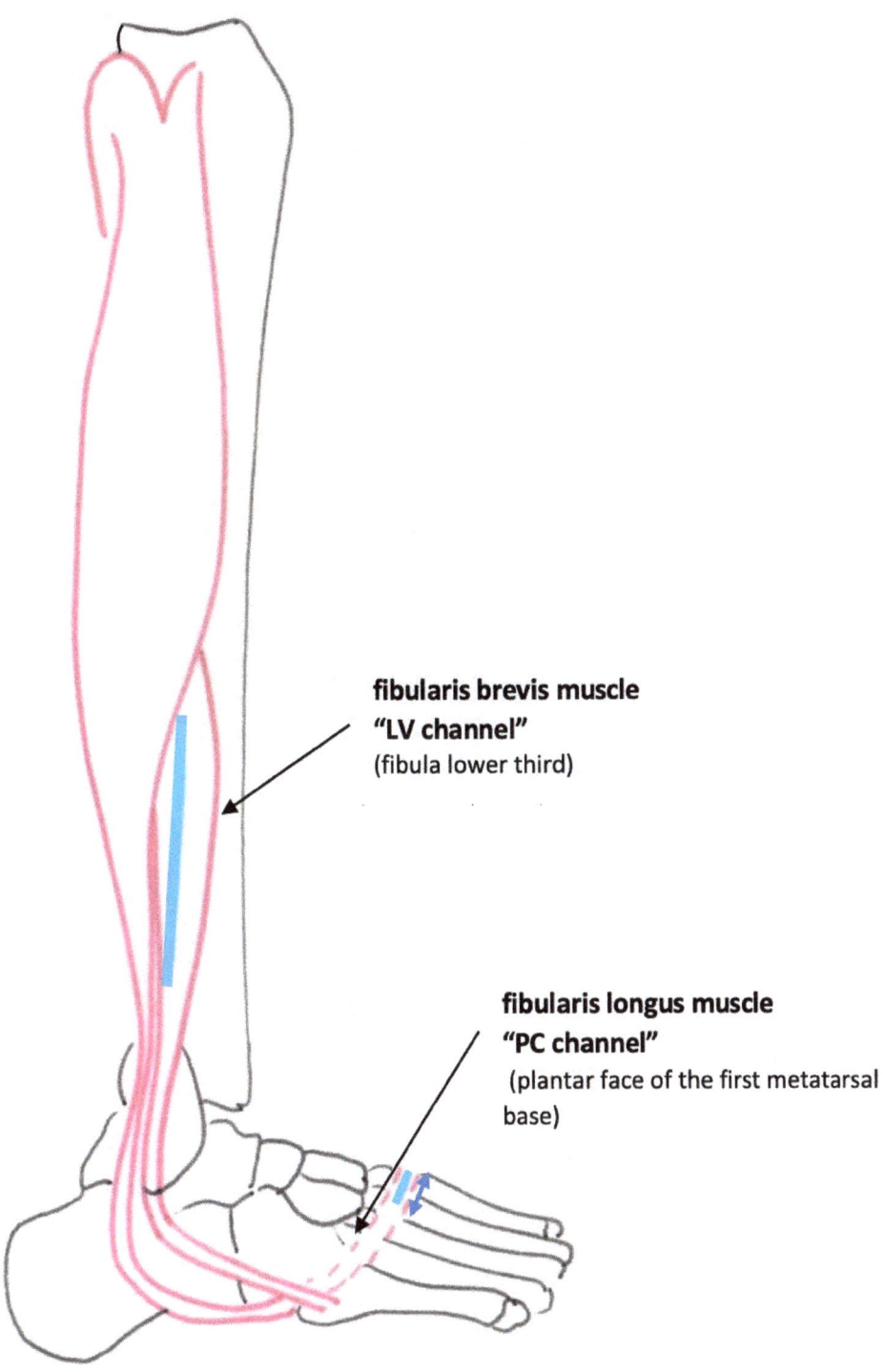

PLATE 4: "LV CHANNEL" "PC CHANNEL" MUSCLES

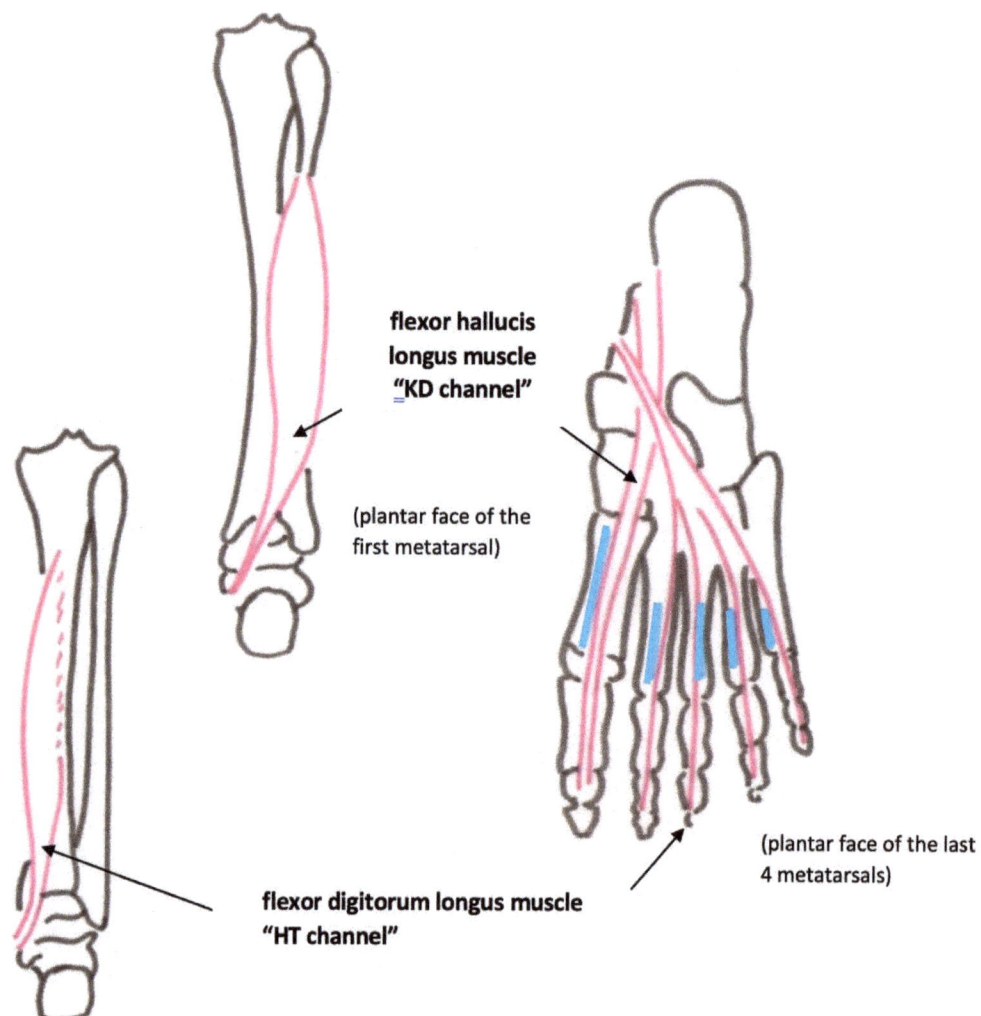

PLATE 5: "KD CHANNEL" "HT CHANNEL" MUSCLES

II – ANATOMICAL DECODING

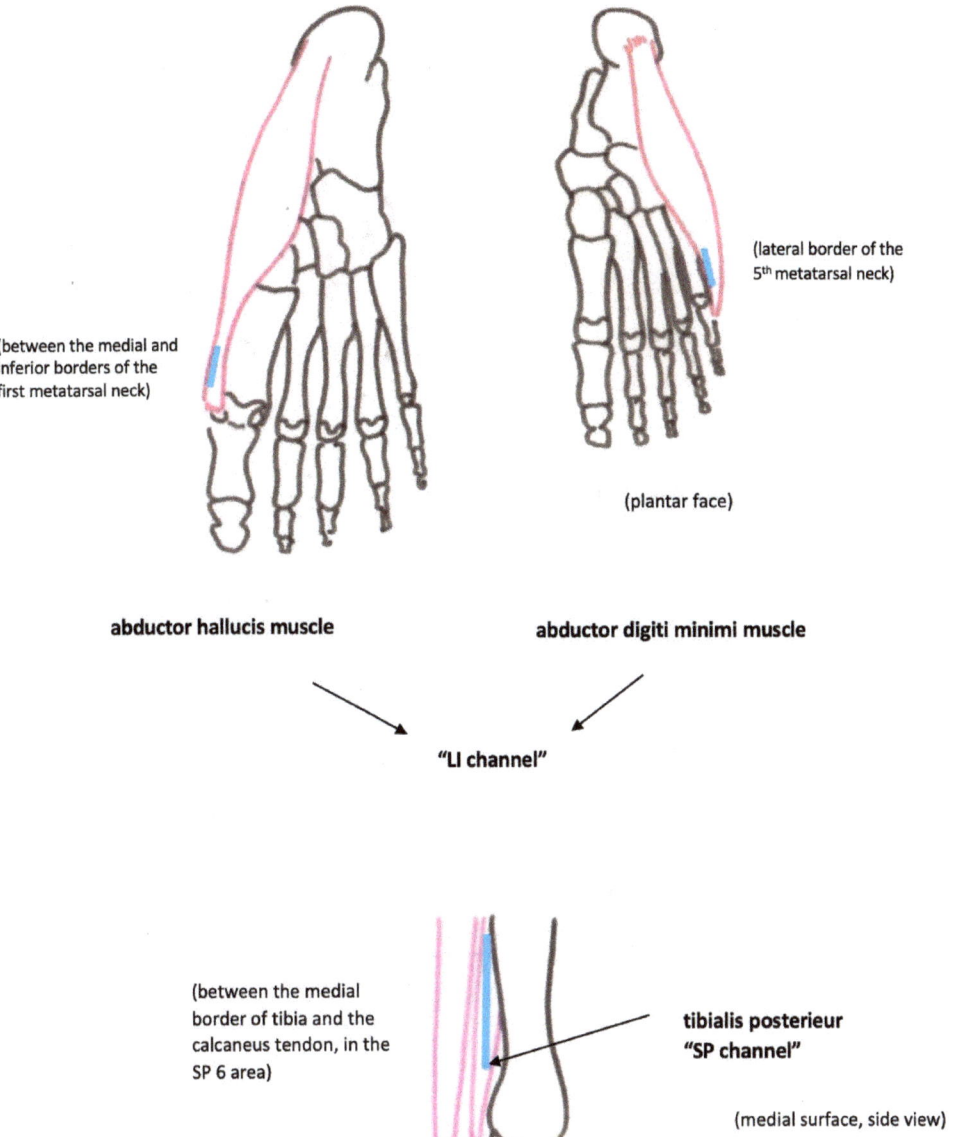

PLATE 6: "LI CHANNEL" "SP CHANNEL" MUSCLES

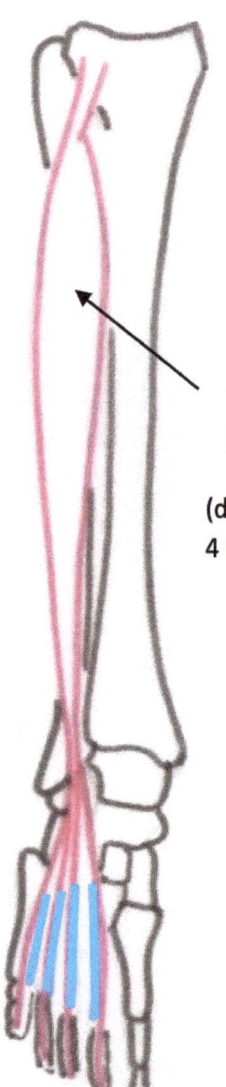

extensor digitorum longus muscle "SI channel"

(dorsal side of the last 4 metatarsals)

fibularis tertius muscle "LU channel"

(lower quarter of the leg, just lateral to the anterior border of tibia)

extensor hallucis longus muscle "UB channel"

(first metatarsal dorsal side)

PLATE 7: "SI CHANNEL" "LU CHANNEL" "UB CHANNEL" MUSCLES

II – ANATOMICAL DECODING

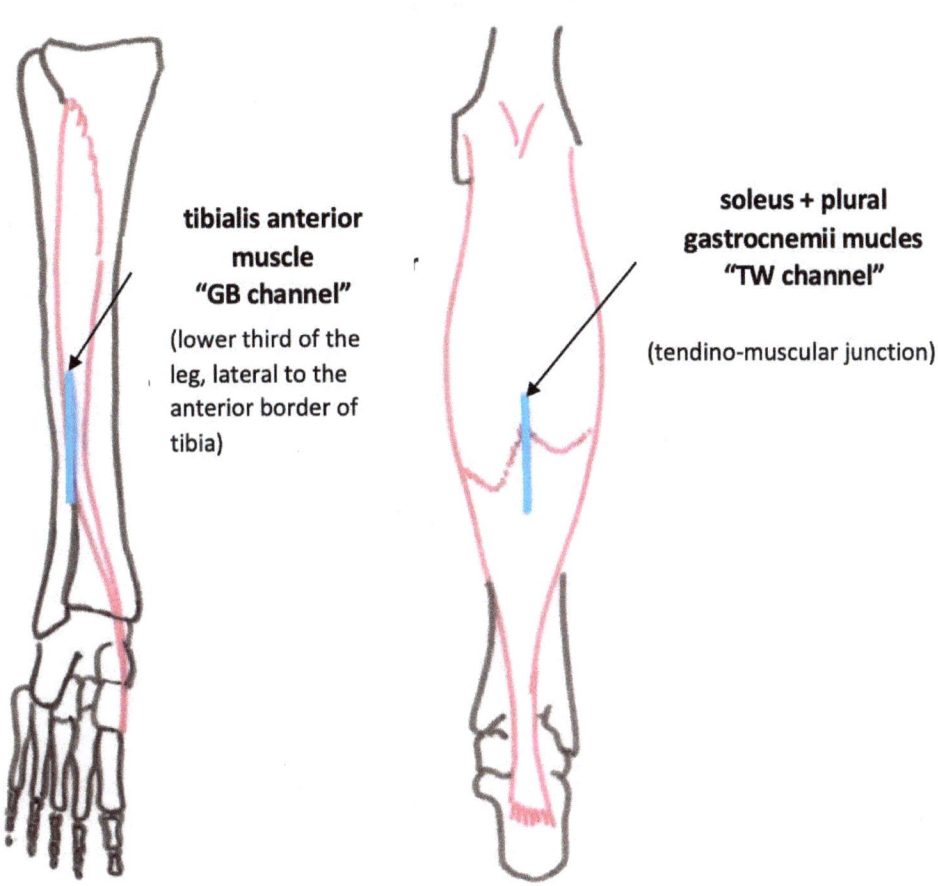

PLATE 8: "GB CHANNEL" "TW CHANNEL" MUSCLES

flexor digitorum brevis muscle "ST channel"

(middle of the plantar face)

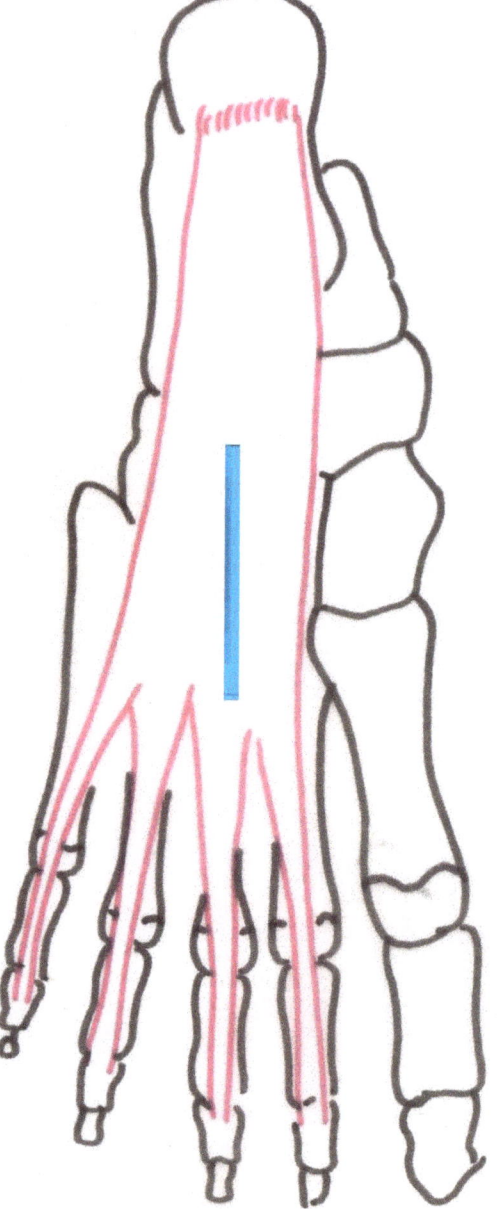

PLATE 9: "ST CHANNEL" MUSCLE

II – ANATOMICAL DECODING

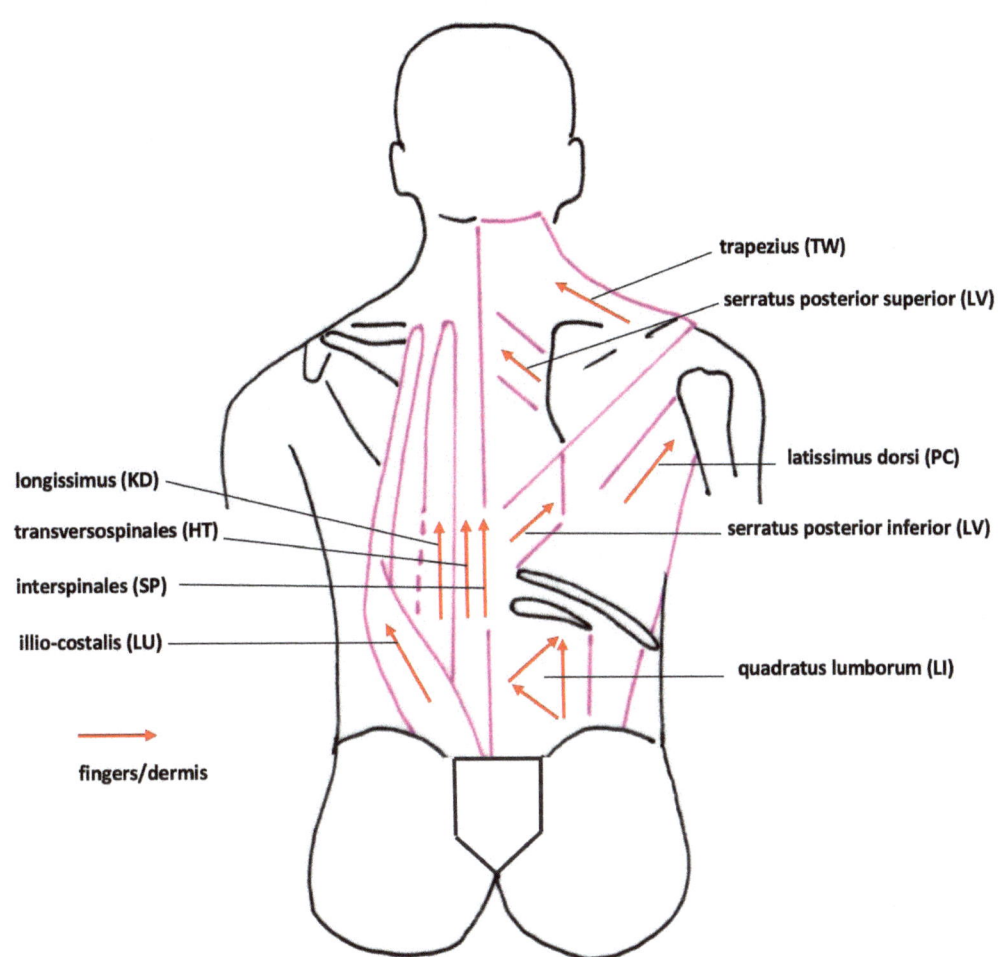

PLATE 10: "ELEMENT" MUSCLES (I)

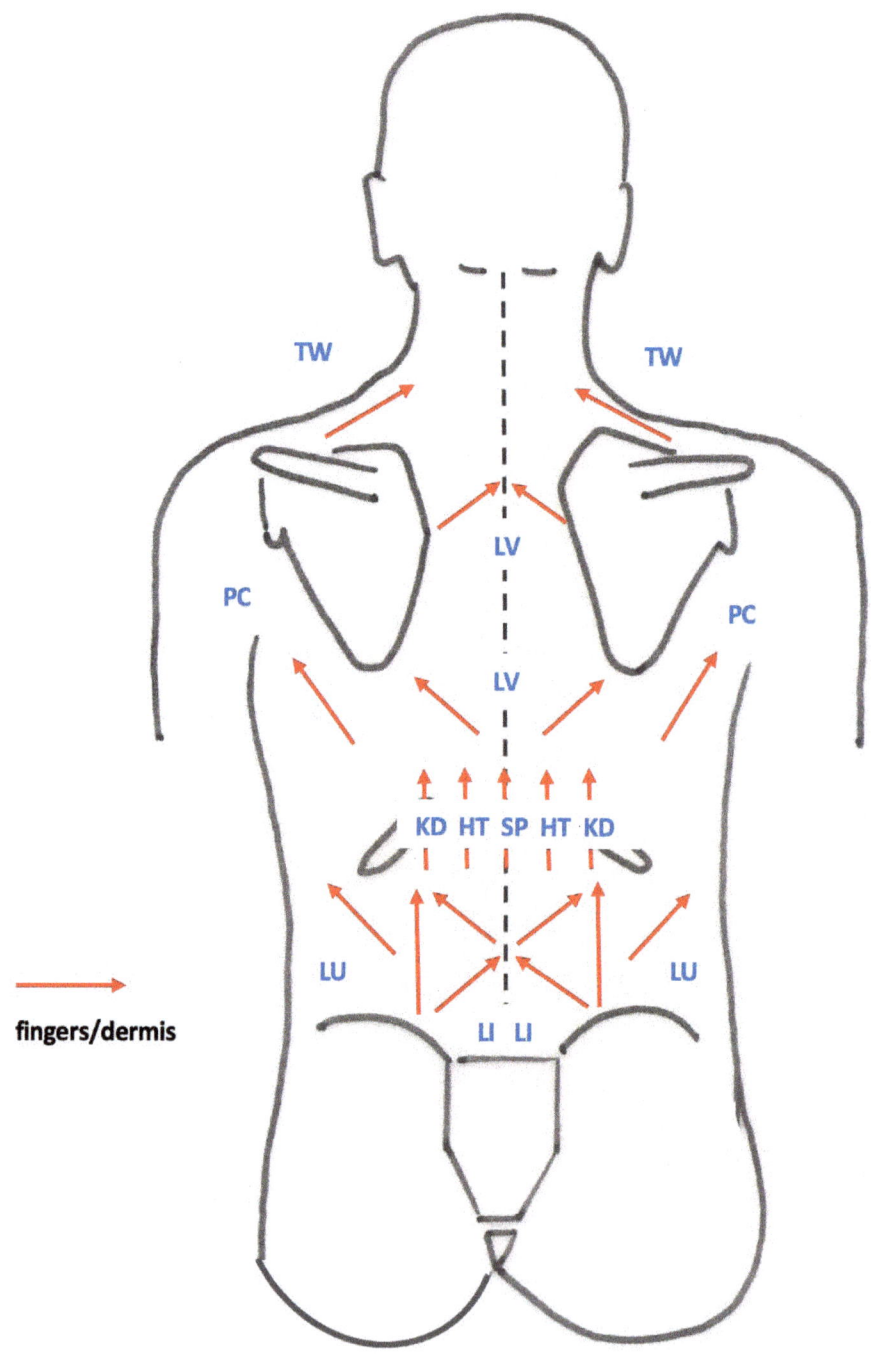

PLATE 11: "ELEMENT" MUSCLES (II)

II – ANATOMICAL DECODING

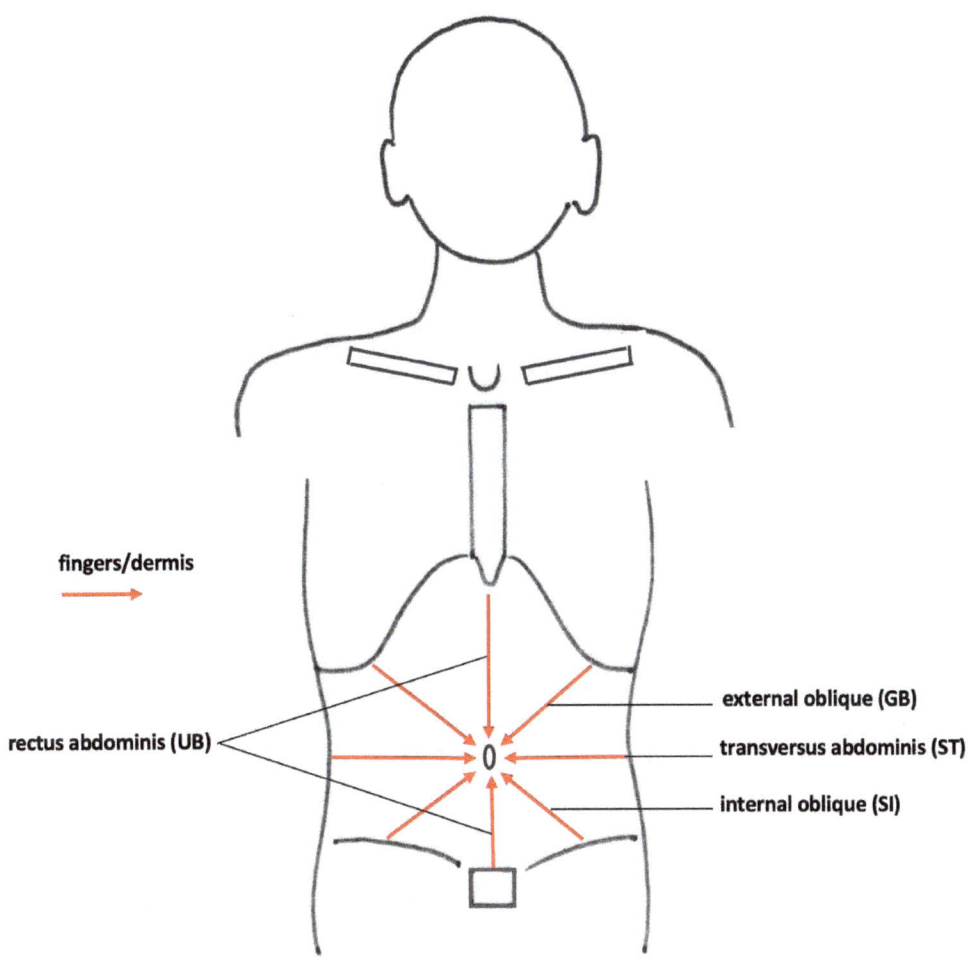

PLATE 12: "ELEMENT" MUSCLES (III)

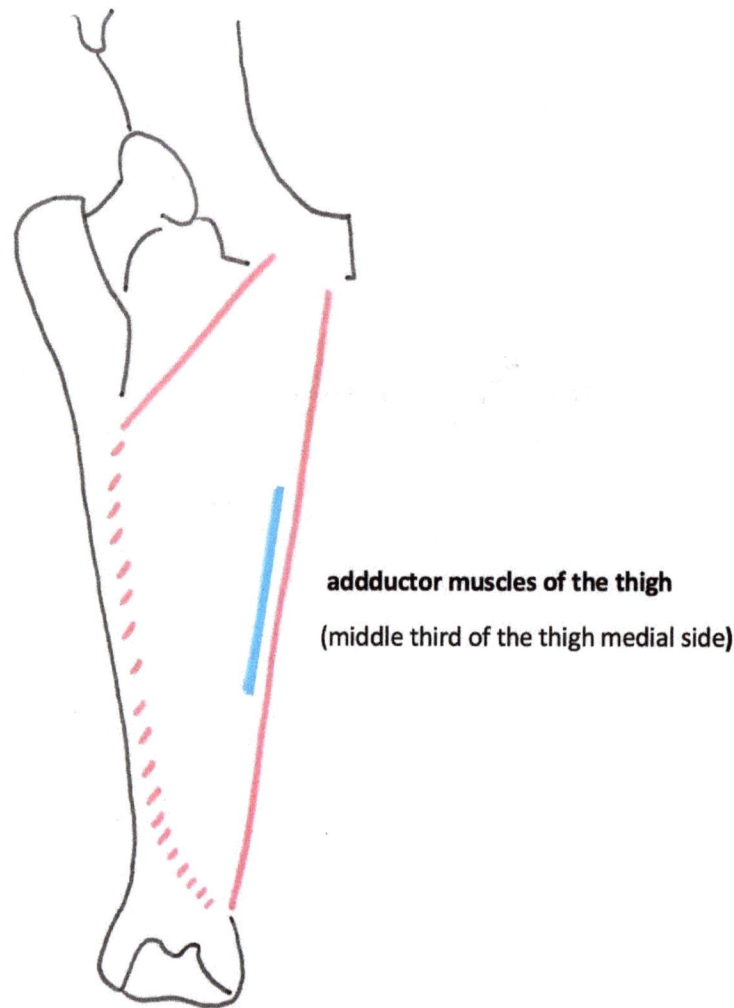

addductor muscles of the thigh

(middle third of the thigh medial side)

PLATE 13: "EXTRAORDINARY CHANNELS" MUSCLES

III – ENERGY MOVEMENT OF THE VISCERA

All body tissues are animated by rhythmic micromovements whose frequency varies according to their embryological origin (endoderm, ectoderm, and mesoderm). Earlier Heaven Qi is the source of this vital rhythm. Passive listening allows to perceive this energy movement which takes the shape, under the hand, of a continuous coming and going, called Primary Respiratory Movement in osteopathy. The frequency for bones and muscles, derived from the mesoderm, is 10 cycles a minute. When the energy does not circulate, this rhythmic swaying disappears, either the therapist has a sensation of stiffness inside the tissue or his hand is always drawn in the same direction.

In order to "listen" to a muscle, the therapist puts his hands down on both its extremities, fingers laid flat crosswise in relation to the longitudinal axis. If the energy circulates in the muscle, he has the sensation that his hands are pulled for 3 seconds in one direction, then 3 seconds backwards (see drawing below).

In order to study the energy movement in the viscera, the practitioner questions

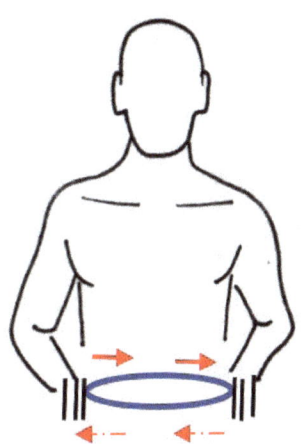

the dermis facing it, in the direction indicated on the plates 14 - 15 which is given by the "migration" (move from one location to another) of the viscera during embryonic development (for example, the stomach rotates 90° clockwise around its longitudinal axis and also rotates clockwise around its antero-posterior axis; the kidneys ascend from the sacral to the lumbar region, at the level of the 12th thoracal vertebra, and rotates medially). It is a faster and more efficient control than passive listening. The energy does not circulate properly in the viscera if the therapist cannot cross the dermis.

These tests give one more indication: whether the energy circulate in such an organ, but it does not indicate the origin of the blockage.

Notes about palpation:
→ As for the organs protected by the ribcage, the palpation is made with the hand palm.
→ Pour As for the viscera (intestines, bladder), it is made with the fingers laid flat.
  → As for the gall bladder and duodenum, palpation is made with both hands using the fingertips.

→ As for the gall bladder, one hand placed within 2 finger breadth above and to the right of the umbilicus, the other hand on the costal margin.

→ As for the duodenum, one hand within 2 finger breadth to the right of the umbilicus, the other hand placed vertically to the first one, below the costal margin.

The sensation of the rope between both hands indicates a blockage of energy in the viscera.

The therapist must make sure the dermis can be mobilized on the underlaying tissue with a usual palpation before interrogating it. The possible blockages must only appear in the direction indicated on the plates.

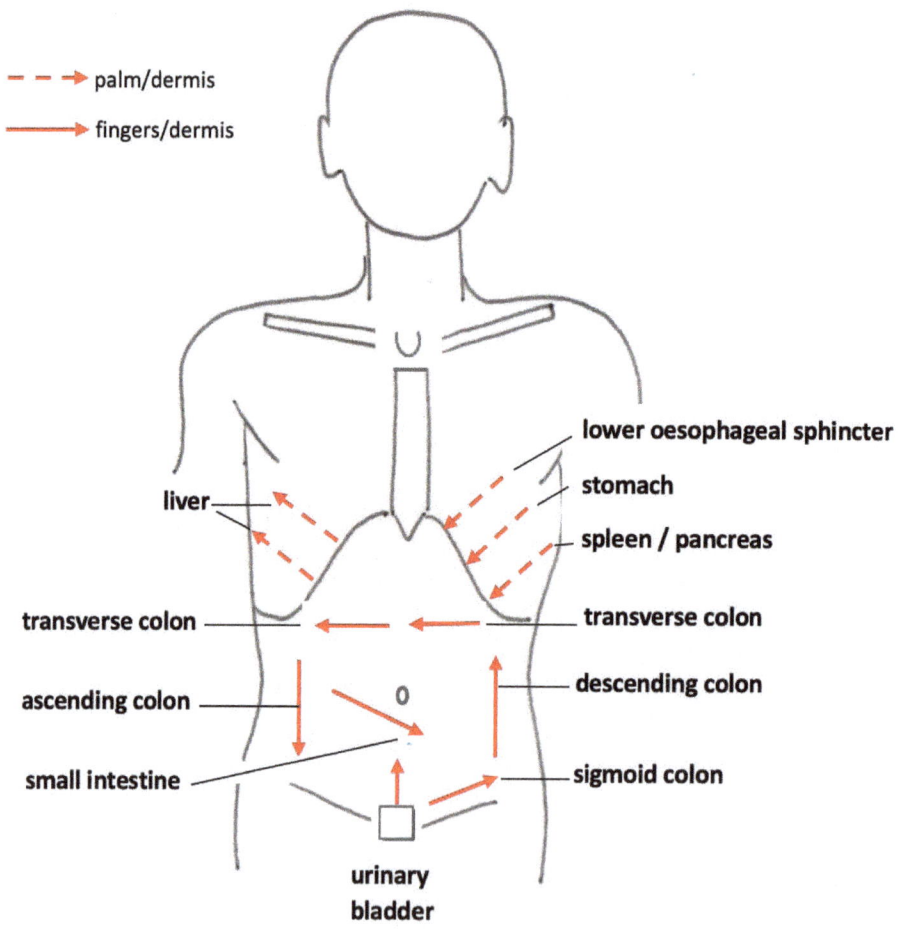

III – ENERGY MOVEMENT OF THE VISCERA

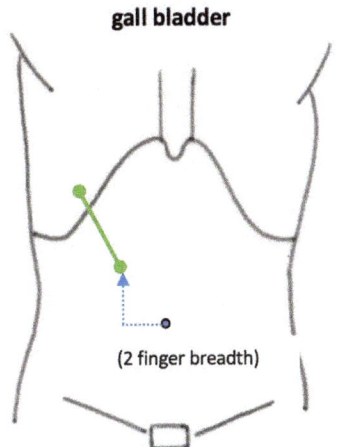

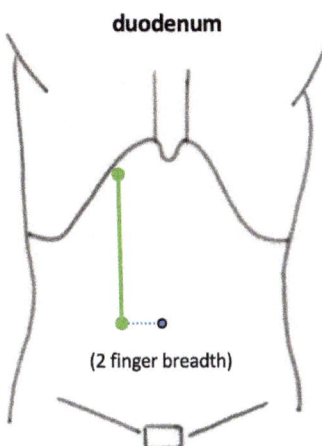

PLATE 14: ENERGY MOVEMENT OF THE VISCERA (I)

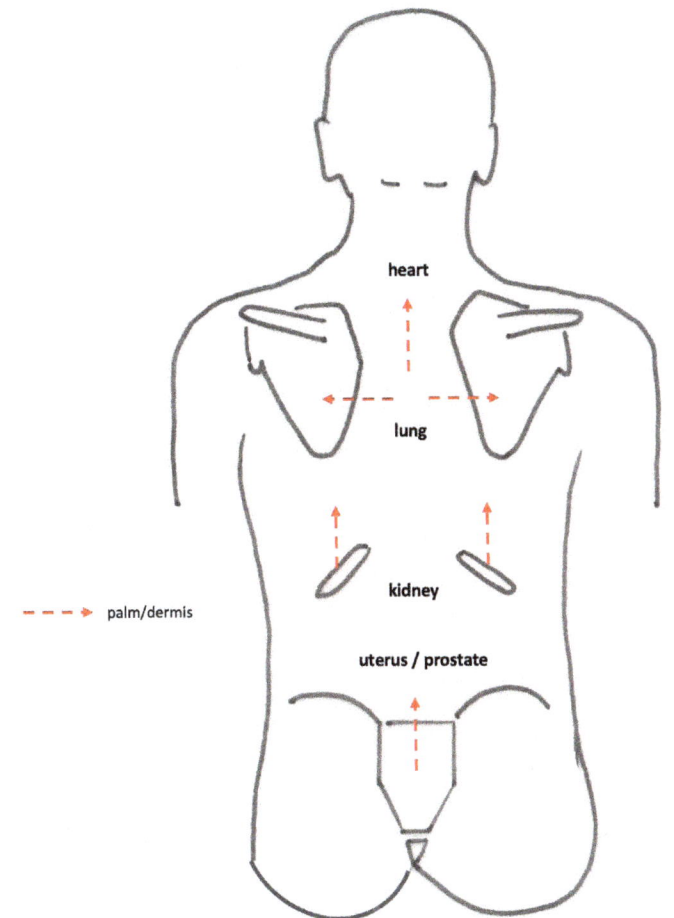

PLATE 15: ENERGY MOVEMENT OF THE VISCERA (II)

IV – THE PHASES OF DISEASE[1]

The morbid development of disease occurs in 6 successive phases, from surface to depth. The seriousness of a pathology is linked to fire penetration which may burn the Yin energy. Its origin is often psychological, therefore emotional chains are important in the treatment.

The 6 phases of disease are related to 6 levels of energetic defence, the 6 paired Channels.

PHASE I: ELIMINATION

Related to the Tai Yang channel (UB – SI)

Water corresponds to the adaptation and elimination capacity. In this phase, the body can first proceed to excretion through the Water of the Urinary Bladder (the Water point and Back-Shu point on the UB channel of each organ and viscera facilitate this function), or otherwise, through the separating Fire of the Small Intestine.

PHASE II: INFLAMMATION (REACTION)

Related to the Yang Ming channel (LI – ST)

The body which cannot eliminate through the Tai Yang, does it through the fire of the Yang Ming.

The Large Intestine is related to the Wei Qi, the Yang defensive energy, and the notion of resistance.

The "square" resistance, which lacks roundness, causes heating and inflammation.

Through the Stomach function, the body can cover with Earth the fire which is rising. If this process goes on, we enter the next phase.

PHASE III: DEPOSITION

Related to the Shao Yang channel (TW – GB)

Toxins that the body could not eliminate, settle in the organs and tissues. It is an

---

1. Jacques Pialoux, *Le Diamant Chauve*, Fondation Cornélus Celsus. Publisher.

encystment phase where benign tumours appear (nodules, warts, mastitis, fibroma, kidney, or gall bladder stones). Note that encystment is a means of protection and that phase III is often more "comfortable" for the patient than phase II.

Related to the Triple Warmer, the Earth Fire is still rising, causing frequent thyroid problems (TW is related to Yang Wei Mai and thyroid). The Gall Bladder can hold back this fire. Chronic stress at work or repressed anger, for example, lead to Qi stagnation in the Gall Bladder which can manifest as symptoms like headaches, red eyes, muscle spasms - neck stiffness, low back pain, tendinitis. The "Weekend Migraines" are often due to the release of accumulated tensions during the workweek (momentary transition from phase III to phase II, i.e., phase of inflammation).

In the Yang phases (the 3 first ones), the diseases are functional and still reversible. From phase IV on, the fire penetrates in depth, the body enters the Yin phases where pathologies are of the "lesional" type.

The Yang phases are of the "excess" type.

The Yin phases are of the "deficiency" type (Yin deficiency in depth).

PHASE IV: IMPREGNATION

Related to the Tai Yin channel (SP – LU)

At this stage, the accumulation of toxins in the organs and tissues leads to chronic diseases as rheumatism, or, in the case of Earth deficiency, chronic inflammatory pathologies (ulcerative colitis, Crohn's disease, inflammatory rheumatism…).

PHASES V: DEGENERATION

Related to the Shao Yin channel (HT – KD)

The Heart Yin deficiency may cause cardiovascular pathologies as hardening of the arteries and high blood pressure, myocardial infarction, stroke, arteritis…

The Heart houses the Shen (Mind). The Empty-Heat generated by Blood and Yin deficiency can disturb the Heart-Shen and lead to mental illness (including mania, burnout, and depression) in severe cases.

The Kidneys nourish Marrow, they are the Root of the Earlier Heaven Qi. At this stage, Kidney Yin is deficient, and Marrow can be affected by the Wei Qi that sinks in deeply causing neurological pathologies (Parkinson's disease, multiple sclerosis…).

PHASE VI: NEOPLASM

Related to the Jue Yin channel (LI – PC)

The fire affects the nucleus of cells that turn toward the energies of the Earlier Heaven and become then immortal.

Appearance of malignant tumours.

Skips are possible from phase II to phase IV, or again from phase III to phase VI after serious physical or emotional shocks (radioactivity, loss, separation…)

The treatment tries to bring back the body toward the elimination phase whenever possible or to achieve a better balance in its phase of disease, tonifying Yin energy and slowing down the fire in the last phases. In all cases, it will be important that the Tai Yang channel functions well and thus, the Back-Shu points and the Du Mai points are open (the Du Mai is linked to the Small Intestine channel through its master point, SI 3). But, as it was mentioned in chapter I, in the corrections to provide, the therapist does not decide anything, he just "listens" to the tissues that show him the disturbed energetic circuits (see chapter XI the centre related to the spleen chain and the phases of disease).

THE READING GRID

→ The Centres
→ Complementary Controls

V – INTRODUCTION TO THE READING GRID

The reading grid has been developed after long palpating observations, some hypotheses were advanced and confirmed by the repetition of these observations on many subjects.

The reading grid indicates to the therapist **where the body is in need**. It determines the therapeutic levels and the energetic functions that are disturbed and require correction. In the manner of a checklist, it is used to control, one by one, the different point categories and channels. Every blockage reflects a disturbance on a given level and is therefore corrected specifically.

The operating mode has been mentioned in chapter I and will be developed further. First, the different controls determine the acupuncture point to be treated in relation to the disturbed function(s). Secondly, the therapist links this point to a precise correction area. He feels as if both his hands were connected by a rope. The sensation is between the hands (and not underneath). He keeps this rope tight and simply waits for its loosening in the following seconds as a sign of self-correction; the point opens at the same time. There is no mechanical action on the point, no tonification nor dispersion. The point's response and communication only matter- "the lack of communication creates the pathology". In fact, the therapist precisely informs the body about the energy disturbance in order to trigger the self-correction mechanism.

There is a fundamental difference between interrogating a tissue with the awareness of the information it bears (what energetic function it is related to) and doing it without that awareness. The response of the tissue under the hand seems stronger and clearer. A well "centred" therapist can sense it first in his abdomen even before putting his hand down and the same holds true when he looks for the correction area.

When interrogating a tissue horizontally, **a blockage which can be interpreted must appear in one precise direction** (as indicated in the previous chapters). Finding it in all directions means that the therapist cannot interpret it according the reading grid (for more explanations, see chapter XXVIII: *Comments on the reading grid*).

V – INTRODUCTION TO THE READING GRID

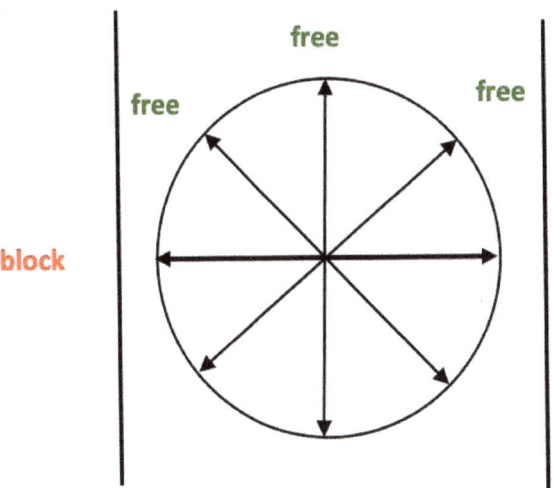

Blockage in a tissue which can be interpreted

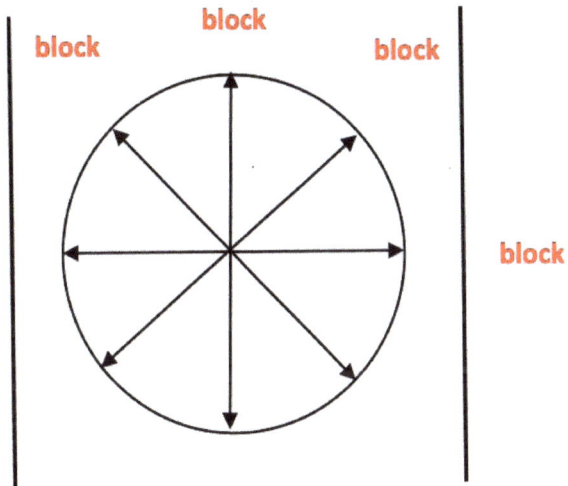

Blockage which cannot be interpreted

In most cases, the interrogation is made horizontally crosswise in relation to the longitudinal axis of the body, the therapist's fingers laid flat. In the description of tests, only the other palpation modes are mentioned (either vertical interrogation or lengthways, or with the hand palm…).

Thus, we shall write:

→ Patella (dermis) for crosswise horizontal interrogation of the dermis in front of the patella, with fingers laid flat.
→ T12 - L1 (palm/surface, lengthways) for horizontal interrogation, with the hand palm, of the T12-L1 vertebral area surface, lengthways.

In the plates we use the following colour code:

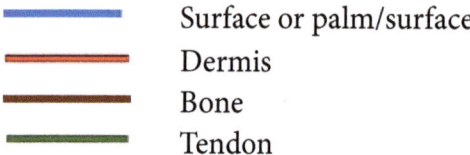

Surface or palm/surface
Dermis
Bone
Tendon

THE CENTRES

- VI — Introduction to the Centres
- VII — Front-Mu Points and Back-Shu Points
- VIII — Emotional Chains of the Du Mai, Stomach, and Gall Bladder Channels
- IX — The Extraordinary Channels
- X — The Specific Centre of the Gall Bladder Channel
- XI — The Specific Centres of the Spleen
- XII — The Specific Centre of the Heart Channel
- XIII — The Occipital Centre
- XIV — The Frontal Centre
- XV — The Physical Trauma
- XVI — The Barriers

VI – INTRODUCTION TO THE CENTRES

The palpatory research has revealed the existence of energetic centres related to the chains of points and the Extraordinary Channels. These centres are both entry doors and correction areas. The chains correspond with the trunk or head part of the lower channels on which the 12 energetic functions are represented as well as the 5 Elements on the peripheral pathway of each channel by the Five Shu points. They are situated on different planes: the inner pathway of the UB channel with the Back-Shu points on the physical plane, the ST or GB chains on the emotional plane, the outer pathway of the UB channel on the spiritual plane.

We find one or several Extraordinary Channels and chains in one centre.

I – PALPATION OF THE CENTRE

The interrogation is horizontal on the surface (= epidermis) with the 4 fingers (except for the thumb) laid flat and placed crosswise in relation to the longitudinal axis.

A blockage indicates at least one disturbed Extraordinary Channel or chain in the centre.

II – DETERMINING THE DISTURBED EXTRAORDINARY CHANNEL OR CHAIN

It is done through the palpation of specific dermis or epidermis areas spread out on the body. Several tests are always possible for each Extraordinary Channel or chain. This allows, on the one hand, to confirm the disturbance that was found and ,on the other hand, since the palpation of an area is not always possible (tissues that cannot be interrogated, bandages, amputation…) to utilize another one that will give the same information.

III – DETERMINING THE DISTURBED ENERGETIC FUNCTION ON THE CHAIN OR EXTRAORDINARY CHANNEL

It is done at the wrist level (and the lower part of the forearm). The energetic functions are located according to the traditional pulse positions of the 5 Elements, but on two levels, of same length - proximal and distal levels (see plate 17). The therapist questions the different tissues (epidermidis, dermis, tendon, or bone) on the whole anterior side of the wrist, with a horizontal palpation, crosswise in relation to the axis of the forearm. The tissue is specific for each Extraordinary Channel or chain. Each point having its own energetic orientation, it is easy to find the one related to the disturbed function. Besides, this point will be closed when palpated. The point/organ decoding are specified in Jacques Pialoux's work[1].

IV – CORRECTION

The correction consists in connecting the blocked point with the centre. The therapist puts one hand slightly on the point, the other one covers the area of the centre until he feels a tight rope between both hands (he ignores the sensation under each hand) and waits for the loosening of the rope. Then, the point is open again and the control areas are blockage free.

If the practitioner is not on the appropriate point, he will not find a rope between this point and the centre.

Notes:

- → The therapist can interrogate one half of a centre located on the mid-line to determine the side of the blockage.
- → The research on the wrist indicates the disturbed Element but not whether it is the organ or the viscera that is affected.
    - → To find it out, the therapist may palpate the related points on the chain or the Extraordinary Channel.
    - → He may also proceed to a mental interrogation. "Energy follows Thought" is a fundamental principle in our practice, already mentioned in the previous chapter. When we "question" a tissue, we do it both with our hands and head.
    - → For instance, the therapist finds through the palpation that a tissue in the Wood position on the wrist is blocked, he then mentally asks if the Liver is affected while questioning the same tissue again. If indeed the Liver is disturbed, the blockage sensation will be equal, even stronger, whereas, if the therapist asks whether the Gall Bladder is affected, it will be less strong or will even disappear.
- → Some centres are linked to a specific organ (Gall Bladder, Heart or Spleen). Blockages caused by physical trauma are treated from the centre located at the ankle.
- → Palpation of tissues and corrections can be easily made through a light piece of clothing.

---

1. Jacques Pialoux, op. cit.

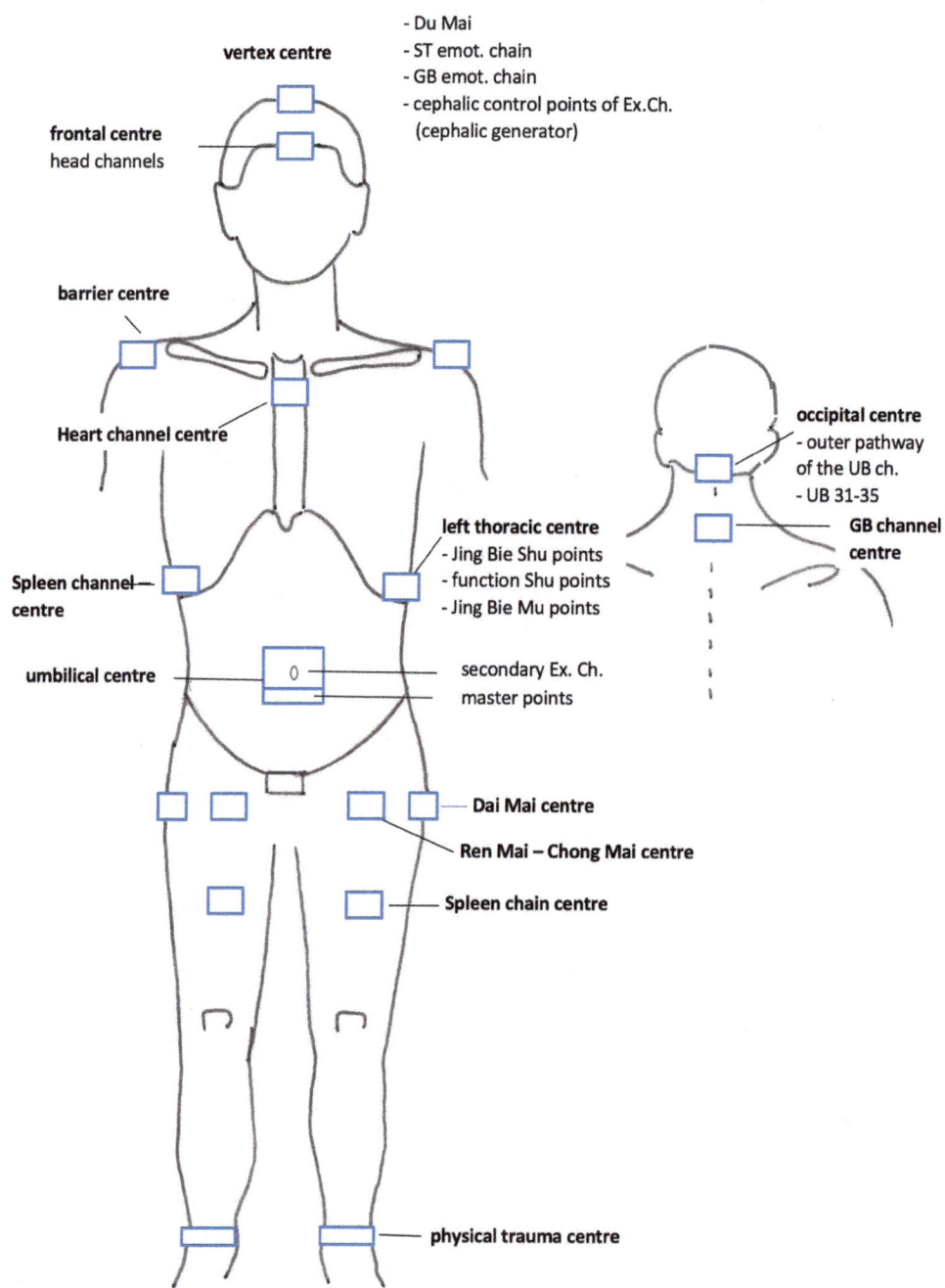

PLATE 16: THE CENTRES

VI – INTRODUCTION TO THE CENTRES

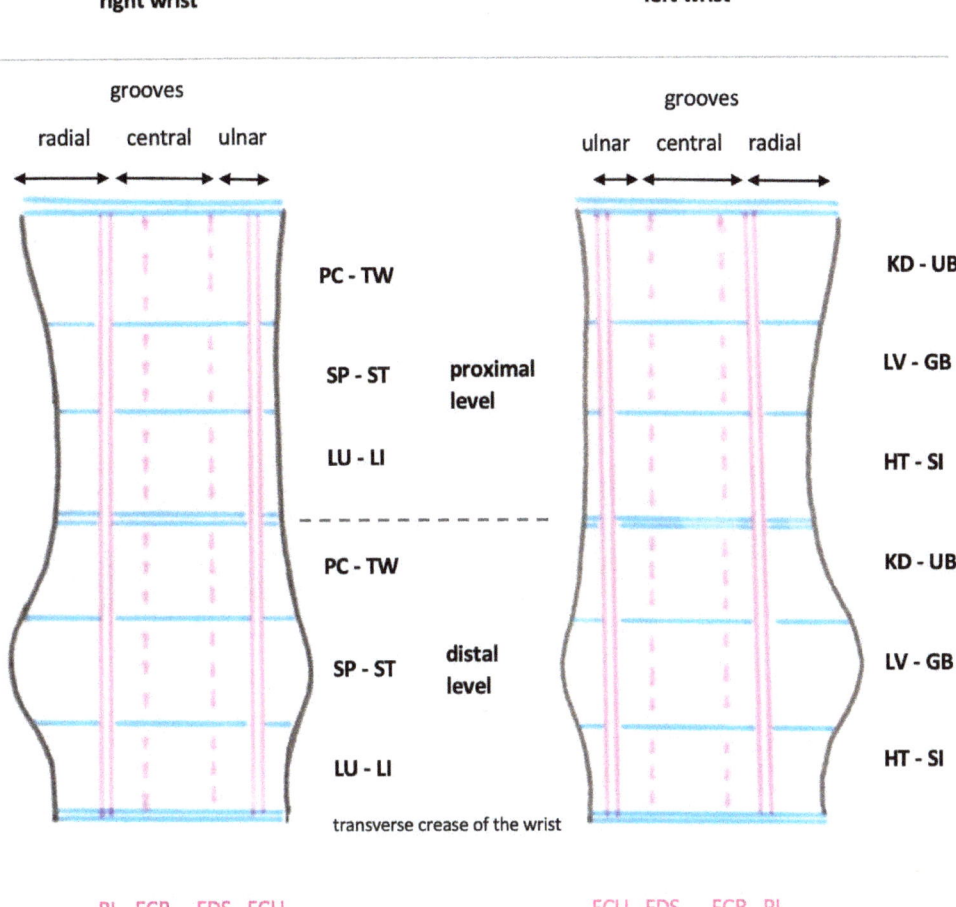

PL = palmaris longus tendon
FCR = flexor carpi radialis tendon
FDS = flexor digitorum superficialis tendon
FCU = flexor carpi ulnaris tendon

PLATE 17: THE ENERGETIC FUNCTIONS AT THE ANTERIOR SIDE OF THE WRIST

VII – FRONT-MU POINTS AND BACK-SHU POINTS

On the inner pathway of the UB channel, Jacques Pialoux distinguishes the classic assent points of organs and viscera, called Jing Bie Back-Shu points, from the function Back-Shu points (great shuttle, wind gate, diaphragm, sea of energy…).

The Jing Bie Back-Shu points, related to the Yang of the organs and viscera, facilitate the elimination of disturbing energies (Xie) coming from external causes (climatic aggressions, toxins, toxic products, infectious agents…) that remain blocked on the surface of the organs and viscera.

(C7) ➡ PC
UB 13 (T3) ➡ LU
UB 15 (T5) ➡ HT
UB 18 (T9) ➡ LV
UB 19 (T10) ➡ GB
UB 20 (T11) ➡ SP
UB 21 (T12) ➡ ST
UB 22 (L1) ➡ TW
UB 23 (L2) ➡ KD
UB 25 (L4) ➡ LI
UB 27 (S1) ➡ SI
UB 28 (S2) ➡ UB

The function Back-Shu points, linked to the 11 points of the Chong Mai (KD 11 ➡ KD 21) that are called function Front-Mu points, tonify Yin energy of the organs and viscera from the depth (they allow the passage of energies from the Chong Mai to the organs and viscera – see chapter IX). Yin deficiency of the Zang organs is more frequent than the one of the Fu organs (viscera).

UB 11 (T1) ➡ KD
UB 12 (T2) ➡ LU
UB 14 (T4) ➡ LV – PC
UB 16 (T6) ➡ HT
UB 17 (T7) ➡ SP
(T8) ➡ ST
UB 24 (L3) ➡ LI

VII – FRONT-MU POINTS AND BACK-SHU POINTS

UB 26 (L5)	➡	SI
UB 29 (S3)	➡	UB
UB 30 (S4)	➡	GB
(coccyx)	➡	TW

The classic Mu points, called Jing Bie Front-Mu points, on the Ren Mai and the front side of the trunk, are rather related to the "3 burner" function (i.e. manufacture of energies) of the organs and viscera. A disturbed Mu point means that the organ (or viscera) itself, as a burner, does not function well.

The Front-Mu points are storage points of acquired Jing Qi (many Front-Mu points belong to the Ren Mai which is the central reservoir of Yin energies) and they serve to tonify the Blood (Yin) of the organs and viscera.

RM 3	➡	UB
RM 4	➡	SI
RM 5	➡	TW
RM 12	➡	ST
RM 14	➡	HT
LV 13	➡	SP
LV 14	➡	LV
GB 24	➡	GB
GB 25	➡	KD
ST 25	➡	LI
LU 1	➡	LU

I – OVERALL CONTROL OF THE 3 LEVELS

➔ Jing Bie Front-Mu
➔ Jing Bie Back-Shu
➔ Function Back-Shu

It is done through the centre located on the lateral side of the left costal margin whether the disturbance is to the left or to the right. As for all centres, the interrogation is horizontal, on the surface, with the fingers laid flat, crosswise in relation to the longitudinal axis of the body. A restriction in the tissue reflects a disturbance in at least one of the 3 levels.

II – DETERMINING THE DISTURBED LEVEL (S)

Several possible tests give the same result for each level. This may be useful to confirm a test or if one of them cannot be done (a tissue that cannot be interrogated...).

- → Jing Bie Front-Mu points
    - → Base of the 3rd metatarsal bone on the dorsal side with a horizontal interrogation, on the surface, crosswise.
    - → Upper front thigh (horizontal interrogation of the dermis, crosswise).
    - → Xyphoid process (lower extremity of the sternum) with a hand palm interrogation, on the surface, lengthways in relation to the body and toward the feet.

- → Jing Bie Back-Shu points
    - → Lateral side of the 5th metatarsal base (surface).
    - → Medial (inner) side of the knee (dermis).
    - → Scapular spine (palm/surface). This test is the same one for the function Back-Shu points.

- → Function Back-Shu points
    - → Mid-transverse crease of the wrist (surface).
    - → Extremity of the medial malleolus and inner side of the astragalus, one finger on each (dermis).
    - → Scapular spine (palm/surface). This test is the same one for the Jing Bie Back-Shu points.

III – DETERMINING THE DISTURBED ENERGETIC FUNCTION

It is done at the wrist level with the palpation of the different Element positions (this test does not indicate whether it is the organ or the viscera in the Element that is disturbed).

- → As for the Jing Bie Front-Mu points, the interrogation is done at the osseous level, in the radial groove, at the proximal level of the wrist. The test is the same one for the function Front-Mu points (Chong Mai – see chapter IX).
- → As for the Jing Bie and function Back-Shu points, the test is identical:

through an interrogation at the dermis level, in the radial groove, at the proximal level of the wrist.

The test is confirmed by the palpation of the related points.
Besides, for the Back-Shu points.

→ Related to the Jing Bie level, the He-Sea point of the disturbed organ or viscera is also closed (it does not respond to a vertical impulse on the surface with the fingertip).
→ Related to the function level, the Yuan-source point is closed.

Rappel:
→ He-Sea points: LU 5 - LI 11 - ST 36 - SP 9 - HT 3 - SI 8 - UB 40 - KD 10 - PC 3 - TW 10 - GB 34 - LV 8
→ Yuan-source points: LU 9 - LI 4 - ST 42 - SP 3 - HT 7 - SI 4 - UB 64 - KD 3 - PC 7 - TW 4 - GB 40 - LV 3

Example:

Let us consider a Liver elimination problem with its Back-Shu point (UB 18) blocked to the right. In this case, we find:
→ A blockage of the centre on the lateral side of the left costal margin.
→ A blockage of the lateral side of the 5th metatarsal base, on the medial side of the knee, on the scapular spine with the previously described palpations, on the right side.
→ A blockage of the dermis of the radial groove, in the Wood position, at the proximal level of the left wrist.
→ The palpation of the points allows to differentiate the Liver or Gall Bladder affliction. In this case the LV 8 point to the right will be closed (not GB 34) as well as the UB 18 to the right (and not UB 19).

IV – CORRECTION

→ Jing Bie Front-Mu points:

The therapist puts down one hand slightly on the affected Mu point and covers with the other hand the area of the centre (at the lateral side of the left costal margin) until he feels a tight rope between both hands, which is essential to trigger off the self-correction.

→ Jing Bie Back-Shu points
   Two steps
   → 1st step: one hand down on the He-Sea point, the other one searches for the rope on the other Shu points (Jing-Well point, Ying-Spring point, Shu-Stream point, Jing-River point) of the same channel, which begins to open up the He point.
   → 2nd step: the therapist keeps one hand down on the He-Sea point, covers the organ or viscera and the related anatomical areas (throat and nose for Lung, pancreas for Spleen, duodenum for Stomach and Gall Bladder…) with the other one in order to find the rope, the loosening of which completely opens the He point. This area corresponds to the imprint of the disturbing agent on the organ or viscera. In the above example, one hand on the LV 8 point, the other one on the liver organ itself.

→ Function Back-Shu points:
   Two steps
   → 1st step: one hand on the Yuan-source point, the other one palpates the 5 Shu points on the same channel searching for the rope, which begins to open the Yuan-source point.
   → 2nd step: the practitioner keeps one hand down on the Yuan-source point and covers the organ or viscera with the other one in order to find the rope.

After the correction, the points respond again and the different tests are blockage free, which is not the case if the correction is incomplete (either the therapist did not quite feel the rope between both hands or he has not waited long enough for its loosening).

Notes:

→ Several blockages of the Shu/Mu points are possible, the palpation process remains the same.
→ The correction of the Back-Shu points is more precise and complete on the organ than on the centre.
→ In the absence of an organ after surgery (spleen, gall bladder, kidney…), the therapist will find the rope anyway in the original location of the organ.

VII – FRONT-MU POINTS AND BACK-SHU POINTS

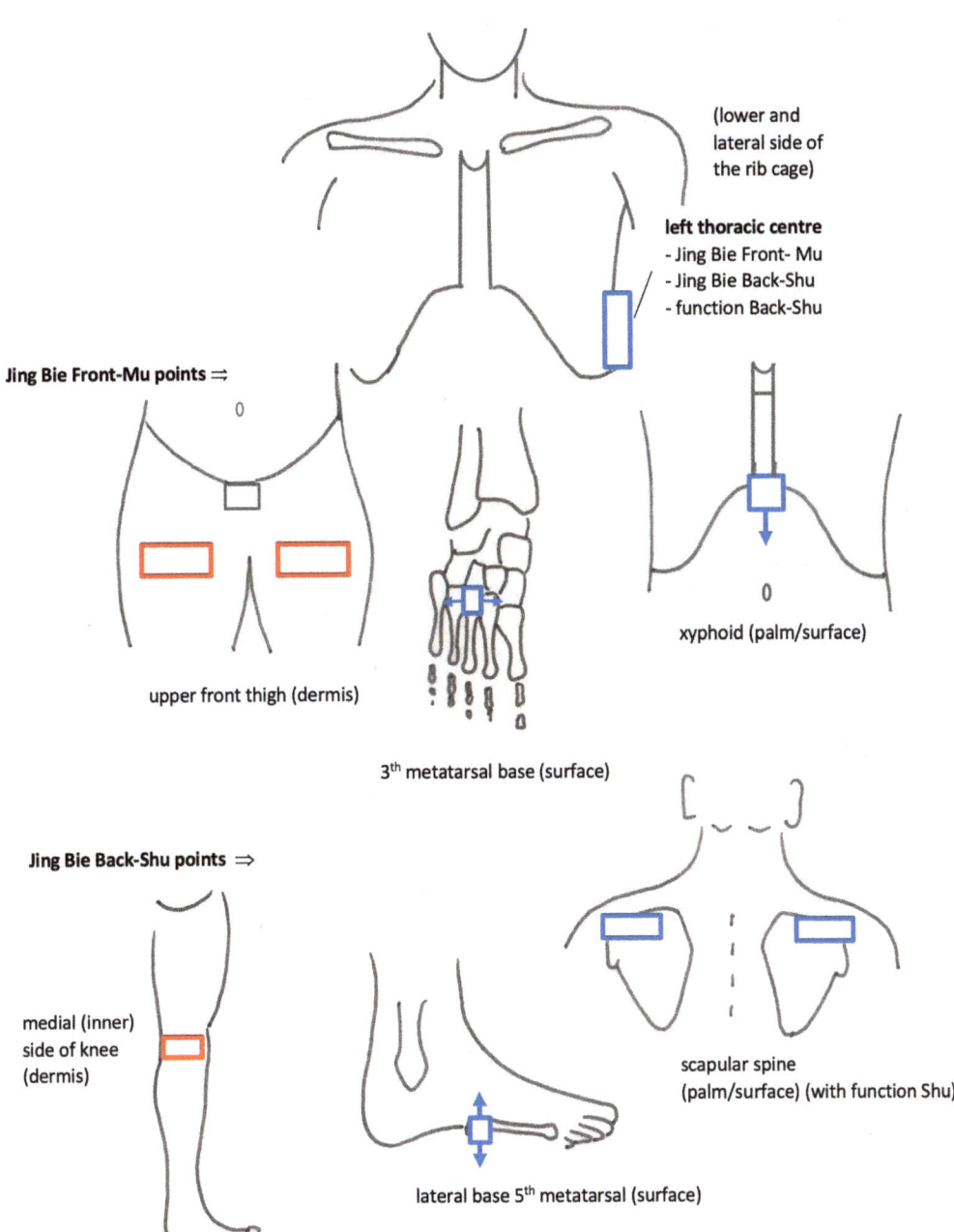

PLATE 18: JING BIE SHU/MU POINTS

Function Back- Shu points ⇒

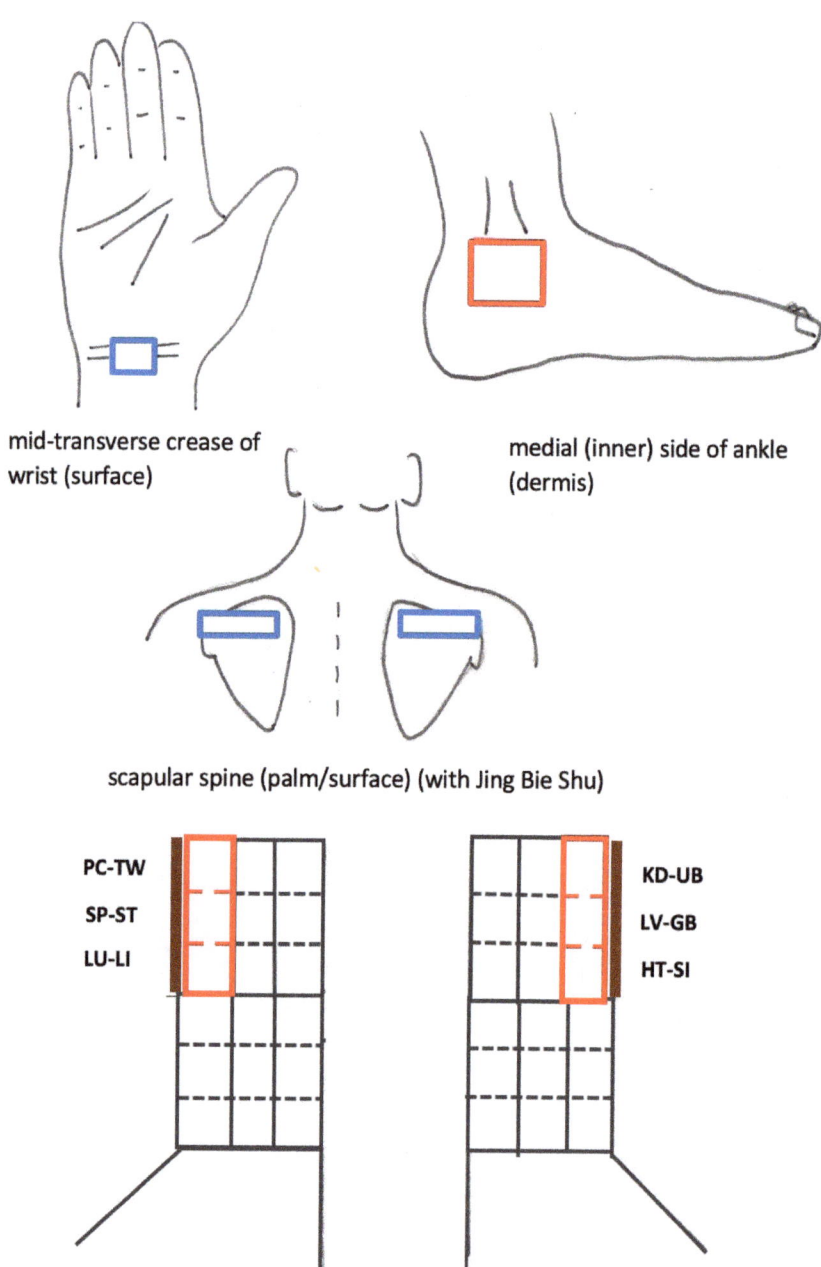

mid-transverse crease of wrist (surface)

medial (inner) side of ankle (dermis)

scapular spine (palm/surface) (with Jing Bie Shu)

PC-TW
SP-ST
LU-LI

KD-UB
LV-GB
HT-SI

Jing Bie Mu (with function Mu) ⇒ proximal radial groove (osseous)

(Jing Bie + function) Shu ⇒ proximal radial groove (dermis)

PLATE 19: JING BIE AND FUNCTION SHU/MU POINTS

VIII – THE EMOTIONAL CHAINS OF THE DU MAI, STOMACH AND GALL BLADDER CHANNELS

Their function is to protect the Heart-Shen from excessive emotions. The vertex centre, at the top of the head, controls both the 3 emotional chains and the cephalic control points of the Extraordinary Channels (cephalic generator).

A – THE EMOTIONAL CHAIN OF THE DU MAI

In the Horary Cycle, at the exit of the Liver channel, the Energy goes up to the brain through the inner pathway of the Liver channel to the DM 20 point, then goes down in the Du Mai and passes in the Ren Mai before entering the Lung channel, at the LU 1 point. The passage through Du Mai and Ren Mai repolarizes the Energy.

The Liver is the major drainer of the energies in the body (it particularly drains the fire from all types of emotions). In case of food and mostly emotional overload, insufficiently purified energies may cause some stagnations in the Du Mai.

Two types of blockage are possible:

→ Function Back-Shu points:
Depending on the nature (Wood, Metal, Water…) of the emotions that turn into fire, some Du Mai points close, either in the vertebral or cranial area.

The most frequent disturbing emotions in relation to the Five Elements:
- → Dissatisfaction, frustration, sense of injustice, resentment cause Liver Qi stagnation which may produce expressed or unexpressed anger. Deficient Wood energy leads to lack of desire, depression (**Wood**).
- → Circular mental rumination, repetitive thoughts may become obsessive, excessive mental work injures the Spleen (**Earth**).
- → Fears (**Water**).
- → Emotional loss, grief, lack of affection (**Fire**) – Blood deficiency and Blood Heat of the Pericardium cause anguish (**Fire Minister**).
- → Sadness, grief, melancholy (**Metal**).

Du Mai decoding

		Vertebral area	Cranial area
Fire minister	➡	DM 14 (C7)	DM 27
Water	➡	DM 13 (T1)	DM 26
Metal	➡	DM 12 (T3)	DM 25
Fire	➡	DM 11 (T5)	DM 24
Fire	➡	DM 10 (T6)	DM 23
Earth	➡	DM 9 (T7)	DM 22
Wood	➡	DM 8 (T9)	DM 21
Wood	➡	DM 7 (T10)	
Earth	➡	DM 6 (T11)	DM 20
Fire minister	➡	DM 5 (L1)	DM 19
Water	➡	DM 4 (L2)	DM 18
Metal	➡	DM 3 (L4)	DM 17
Wood	➡	DM 2 (S4)	DM 16

Notes:

→ A fire related to Metal, which has been insufficiently drained by the Liver, can lead to a stagnation at DM 3 and DM 12 ("Metal points") on the vertebral pathway of Du Mai or at DM 17 and DM 25 ("Metal points") on the cranial pathway
→ In energy circulation: a local obstruction on the Du Mai pathway.

I - OVERALL CONTROL OF THE DU MAI

Several tests are possible:

→ 2nd phalanx of the thumb in crosswise interrogation at the osseous level.
→ Sacrum in crosswise interrogation (dermis).

II – DETERMINING THE DISTURBED VERTEBRAL OR CRANIAL AREA

Interphalangeal (IP) thumb articulation (surface) ➡ cranial part (resonance blockage) 2nd phalanx (P2) of the thumb, below the nail (surface) ➡ vertebral part (resonance and circulation blockages)

➔ Sacrum (palm/surface) ➡ cranial part (resonance blockage.
T12 - L1 area: (palm/surface) ➡ vertebral part
either crosswise ↕ resonance blockage
or lengthways ↔ circulation blockage

To sum up:

P2 pouce (os)
↗ cranial Du Mai = IP thumb (surface) (resonance)
↘ vertebral Du Mai = P2 thumb (surface) (resonance and circulation)

Sacrum (derme)
↗ cranial Du Mai = sacrum (palm/surface) (resonance)
    crosswise ↔ = resonance
    ↗
↘ vertebral Du Mai = T12 – L1 (palm/surface)
    ↘
    lengthways ↕ = circulation

III – DETERMINING THE DISTURBED ENERGETIC FUNCTION (IN RESONANCE BLOCKAGE)

It is done at the distal level of the wrist, according to the 5 Element positions.

As for the cephalic Du Mai, the practitioner questions the surface (= epidermis) in the radial groove.

As for the vertebral Du Mai, he questions the palmaris longus tendon with a crosswise impulse: he can either penetrate the tendon or on the contrary bumps against a rope that is too tight.

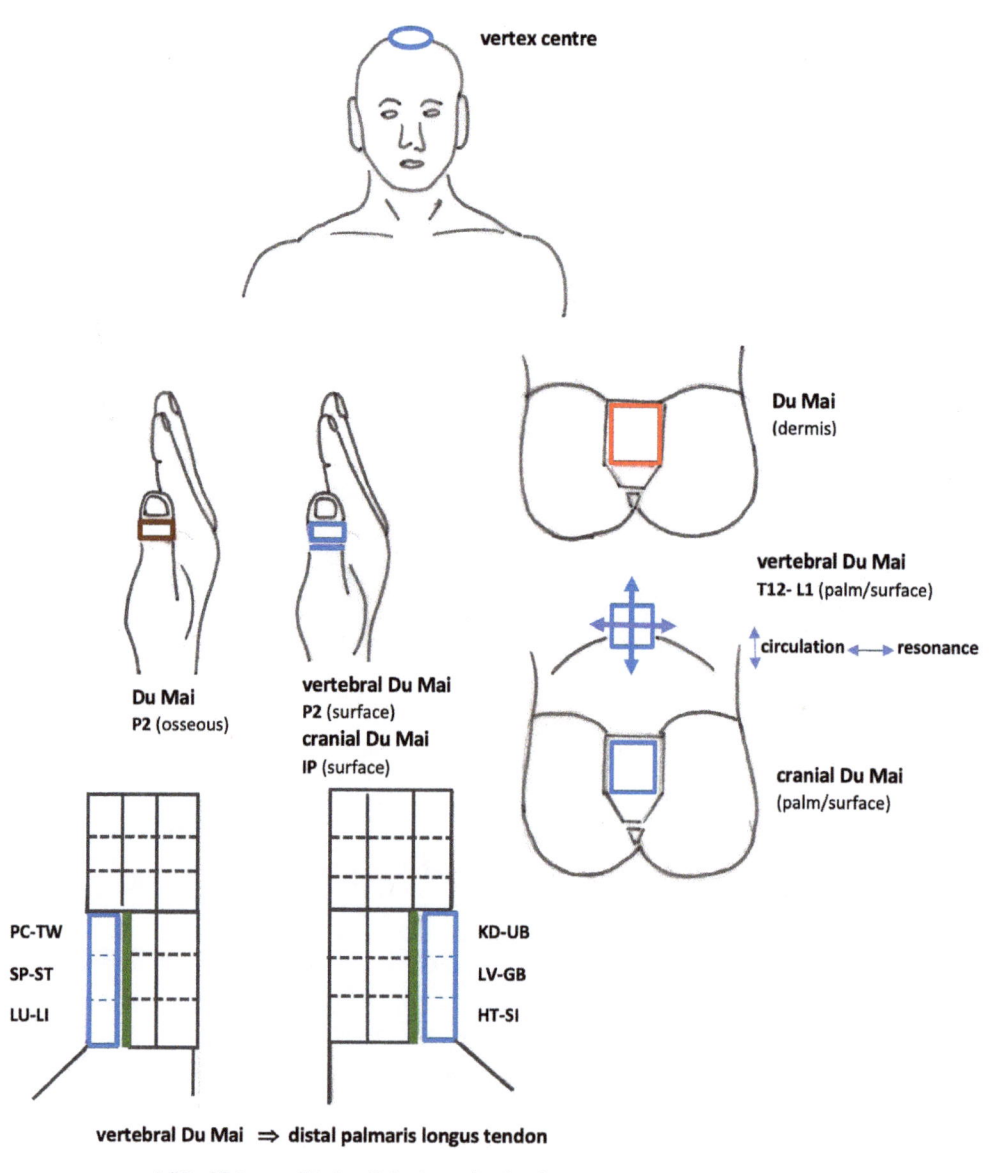

PLATE 20: EMOTIONAL CHAIN OF THE DU MAI

VIII – THE EMOTIONAL CHAINS OF THE DU MAI, STOMACH AND GALL BLADDER CHANNELS

Confirmation:
→ through the palpation of the related points on the Du Mai.
→ through the palpation of the 5 Shu points of the Liver channel.

For instance, if the Water position at the tendon level or on the surface is not free, LV 8 point (Water point) is closed on the blocked side in the overall control (thumb P2 or hemi-sacrum).

IV – CORRECTION

→ Concerning resonance blockages: one hand on the Du Mai point, the other one covers the vertex area (top of the head) until the therapist finds the rope between both hands.
→ Concerning circulation blockages at the vertebral level, the practitioner strokes the spine with his fingertips till he feels an obstacle that keeps his hand from sliding (here, once again, the sensation is not only under the hand but also in the abdomen). The therapist strokes this area 2 or 3 times until the bumping sensation disappears.

B – THE EMOTIONAL CHAIN OF THE STOMACH CHANNEL

When the Liver can no longer drain the emotions that turned into fire, the Pericardium intervenes to protect the Heart. This fire overheats the Pericardium which drains off on the Stomach chain from ST 11 to ST 30, the Stomach being the PC's emunctory through its midday/midnight relationship with the PC. Most emotional shocks are imprinted on this chain (ST 14 is a major point, often blocked after any kind of emotional shock).

The decoding follows the one of the inner pathway of UB channel. The points that have the same numeration as the Jing Bie Back-Shu points are related to the organ surface, the points that have the same numeration as the function Back-Shu points are related to the organ depth.

ST 11 ➡	Water	KD
ST 12 ➡	Metal	LU
ST 13 ➡	Metal	LU
ST 14 ➡	Wood-Fire Minister	LV-PC
ST 15 ➡	Fire	HT
ST 16 ➡	Fire	HT

ST 17 ➡	Earth	SP
ST 18 ➡	Wood	LV
ST 19 ➡	Wood	GB
ST 20 ➡	Earth	SP
ST 21 ➡	Earth	ST
ST 22 ➡	Fire-Minister	TW
ST 23 ➡	Water	KD
ST 24 ➡	Metal	LI
ST 25 ➡	Metal	LI
ST 26 ➡	Fire	SI
ST 27 ➡	Fire	SI
ST 28 ➡	Water	UB
ST 29 ➡	Water	UB
ST 30 ➡	Wood	GB

Example:
➡ An excessive fear may close ST 11 and ST 23 ("KD points").

I – OVERALL CONTROL OF THE STOMACH EMOTIONAL CHAIN

Several tests are possible:
➡ Pisiforme (surface)
➡ Patella (dermis)
➡ Pectoral region, above the nipple (palm/surface, the impulse is directed downwards, toward the feet).

II – DETERMINING THE DISTURBED ENERGETIC FUNCTION

It is done at the proximal level of the wrist, on the surface, in the radial groove.

Confirmation:
➡ Through the palpation of the related points of the stomach chain.
Example: If the Fire position is not free, the therapist palpates ST 15, ST 16 ("HT points") and ST 26, ST 27 ("SI points") on the blocked side in the overall control and keeps the one that does not respond.
➡ Through the palpation of the Shu points on the PC channel. In the above example, PC 8 (= Fire point) is closed on the same side.

III – CORRECTION

The therapist's one hand on the point of the Stomach chain, the other one covers the vertex area to find the rope.

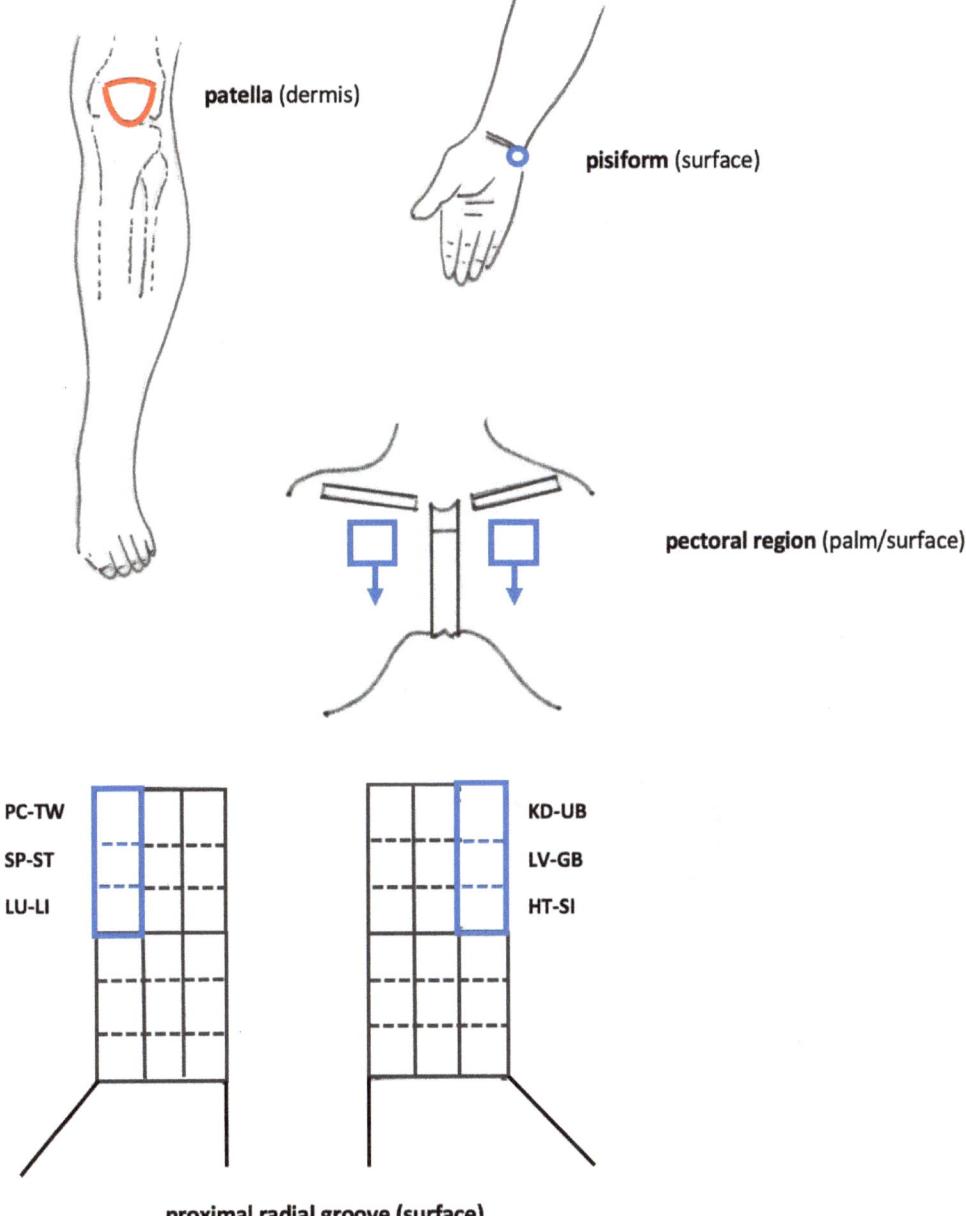

PLATE 21: EMOTIONAL CHAIN OF THE STOMACH CHANNEL

C – THE EMOTIONAL CHAIN OF THE GALL BLADDER CHANNEL

If the Liver Yang, fed by the fire of emotions, rises and the Pericardium is overworked, the Gall Bladder can hold back the Liver energy to keep it from passing into the Heart (whereas, physiologically, the Gall Bladder channels the Liver movement and gives it its direction toward the Heart). This results in Qi stagnation or excess heat in the Gall Bladder. Most of the unexpressed emotions are imprinted on the GB channel.

Two levels to consider:

Trunk level

GB 22 ➡	Metal	LU
GB 23 ➡	Fire	HT
GB 24 ➡	Wood	GB
GB 13 ➡	Earth	SP
GB 14 ➡	Wood	LV
GB 25 ➡	Water	KD
GB 26 ➡	Fire Minister	TW
GB 27 ➡	Earth	ST
GB 28 ➡	Metal	LI
GB 29 ➡	Fire	SI
GB 30 ➡	Water	UB

Cranial level

GB 9 (Tianchong) ➡	Earth	ST
GB 10 ➡	Fire Minister	TW
GB 11 ➡	Metal	LI
GB 12 ➡	Water	KD
GB 14 ➡	Metal	LU
GB 15 ➡	Fire	HT
GB 16 ➡	Wood	LV
GB 17 ➡	Wood	GB
GB 18 ➡	Earth	SP
GB 19 ➡	Fire	SI
GB 20 ➡	Water	UB

VIII – THE EMOTIONAL CHAINS OF THE DU MAI, STOMACH AND GALL BLADDER CHANNELS

GB 1 to GB 8 and GB 13 (Benshen, GB 9 in a former nomenclature) will be studied in relation to the Extraordinary channels (cephalic psychosomatic generator level) and the Heart channel).

I – OVERALL CONTROL

- → Trunk level
    - → Patella tendon (dermis).
    - → Lateral side of the thoracic cage (palm/surface lengthways).
- → Cranial level
    - → Patella tendon (surface).
    - → Anterior side of the shoulder (palm/surface, the impulse is given downwards, toward the feet).

II – DETERMINING THE DISTURBED ENERGETIC FUNCTION

It follows the same process as previously described for the other chains.
- → At the distal level of the wrist:
    - → Trunk level: flexor carpi ulnaris tendon.
    - → Cranial level: ulnar groove (surface).

Confirmation:
- → Through the palpation of the related point on the GB chain.
- → Through the palpation of the related Shu points (Wood, Fire, Water… points) on the GB channel.

III – CORRECTION

The therapist puts one hand on the closed point of the GB chain (trunk or cranial levels), the other hand on the vertex centre.

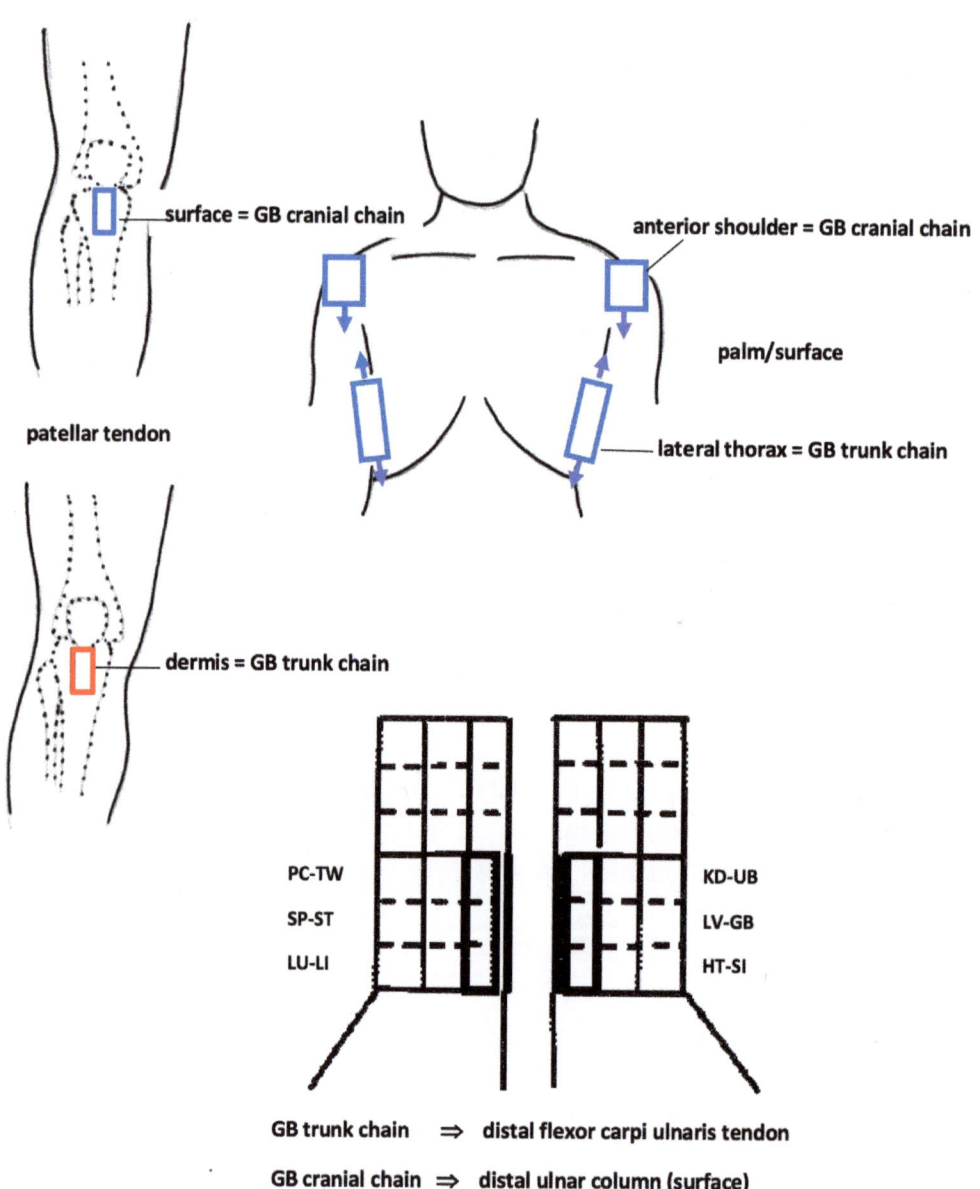

PLATE 22: EMOTIONAL CHAIN OF THE GALL BLADDER CHANNEL

D – OVERALL CONTROL OF THE 3 EMOTIONAL CHAINS (DU MAI-STOMACH-GALL BLADDER) ON THE METATARSAL DORSAL SIDE

It is done through a horizontal palpation, lengthways, on the surface.

Decoding is identical to the one of the hand:

- M1 ➡ Earth
- M2 ➡ Metal
- M3 ➡ Water
- M4 ➡ Wood
- M5 ➡ Fire – Fire Minister

Example:

➔ A 3rd metatarsal blockage to the right indicates a disturbance of the Water points (KD or UB) in at least one of the three chains to the right.

E – OVERALL CONTROL: THE VERTEX CENTRE

We do remind that the three emotional chains can be controlled globally at the vertex centre level which also includes the cephalic psychosomatic generator (= cephalic control points of the Ex. Ch.).

A vertex blockage to the right indicates a disturbance of an energetic function in at least one of the three emotional chains or in the cephalic generator, to the right.

IX – THE EXTRAORDINARY CHANNELS[1]

The 3 burners produce 2 energies (the one, nutritive, Yin, the other, defensive, Yang). The 8 Extraordinary Channels distribute these energies to the 11 organs/viscera and the 12 channels which will utilize them. The Chong Mai points and the master points allow in particular to control this distribution.

The Extraordinary Channels are like an immense reservoir with 8 compartments which contribute to regulate the flow of Qi and Blood in the regular channels and throughout the body, in the different planes of space.

→ Depth/surface ➡ Chong Mai/Dai Mai axis
→ Front/back ➡ Ren Mai/Du Mai axis
→ Right/left ➡ Yin Qiao Mai/Yang Qiao Mai axis
→ Lower/upper ➡ Yin Wei Mai/Yang Wei Mai axis

That is how, for instance, the Energy is on the surface in case of Chong Mai deficiency.

The constituent points of the Ex.Ch. are also utilized to eliminate the disturbing energies in the main channels locally.

The 4 main, central Extraordinary Channels are coupled with the 4 secondary Ex.Ch.:
→ Chong Mai coupled with Yin Wei Mai
→ Ren Mai coupled with Yin Qiao Mai
→ Du Mai coupled with Yang Qiao Mai
→ Dai Mai coupled with Yang Wei Mai

The paired Extraordinary Channels support one another.

The Extraordinary Channels are the link between the Earlier Heaven and the Later Heaven. They allow the passage of the Earlier Heaven energies (stored in Kidneys and Extraordinary Yang organs: brain, bone marrow, uterus, gall bladder…) towards the organs of the Later Heaven (Spleen, Liver, intestines …), hence their resonance with the endocrine glands. A disturbance at their level, often caused by emotional trouble, can result in hormonal disorders.

Chong Mai is in resonance with the hypothalamus.

---

1. For a more extensive theoretical study, see J. PIALOUX's work, "Le Diamant Chauve Plus".

Yin Wei Mai	➡	Gonads
Yin Qiao Mai	➡	Adrenal glands
Ren Mai	➡	Thymus
Du Mai	➡	Epiphysis
Yang Qiao Mai	➡	Hypophysis
Yang Wei Mai	➡	Thyroid – parathyroid glands
Dai Mai	➡	Endocrine pancreas

A – THERAPEUTIC LEVELS AND CENTRES

There are 3 levels to consider:

- The Extraordinary Channels with their constituent points.
- The master points.
- The cephalic psychosomatic generator (points from GB 1 to GB 9 - actual GB 13).

These 3 levels appear on the hand:

- The thumb column = the Extraordinary Channels with their constituent points.
- Interphalangeal articulations of the fingers = the 8 master points.
- Head and base of the finger metacarpal bones = the cephalic generator.

The centres:

- Chong Mai and Ren Mai on the anterior upper thigh.
- Dai Mai on the greater trochanter.
- Du Mai and the cephalic generator on the vertex (with ST and GB emotional chains).
- The secondary Ex.Ch. and the master points on the umbilical centre: 5 horizontal stripes, one finger breadth, and one index finger length, on each side of the umbilicus.

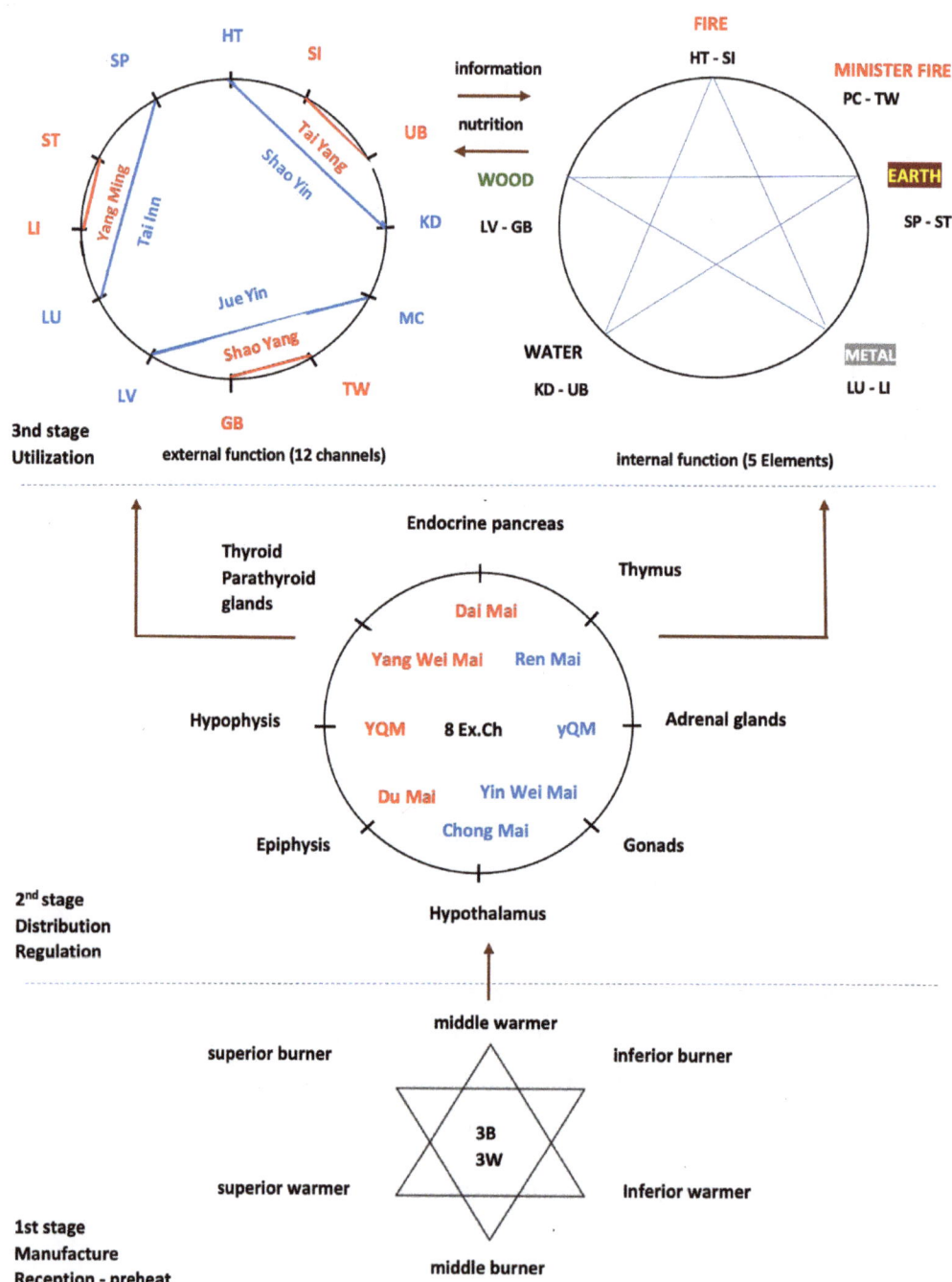

PLATE 23: THE 3 STAGES OF THE ENERGETIC SYSTEM
(according to J. PIALOUX)

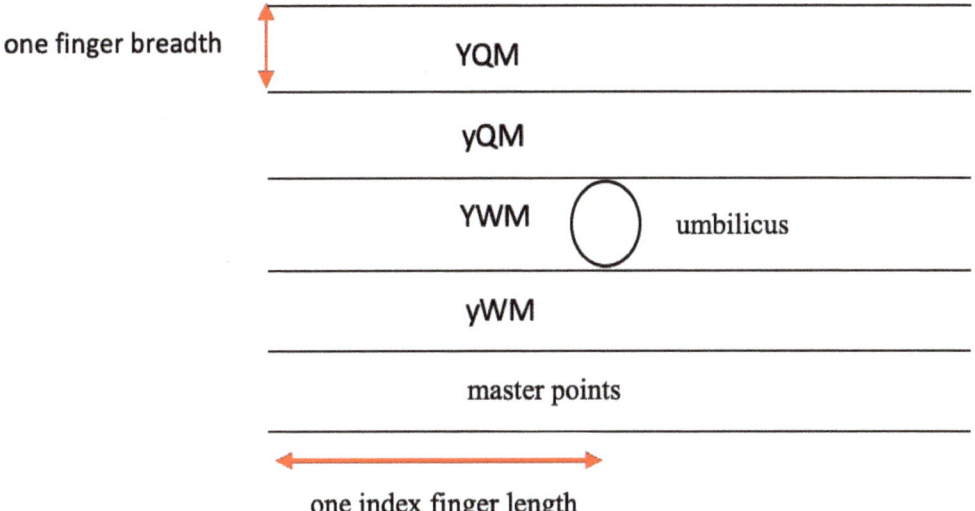

Note:

→ If Ren Mai and Du Mai are blocked only in circulation, their disturbance does not appear at the centre level.

B - THE CENTRAL EXTRAORDINARY CHANNELS

REN MAI (central reservoir of Yin energies)

The congenital Jing Qi and the extra acquired Jing Qi, which is not being used, are stored in the Kidneys and Ren Mai.

I - OVERALL CONTROL

→ First phalanx (P1) of the thumb (osseous) with the upper burner – middle burner – lower burner from its head to its base.

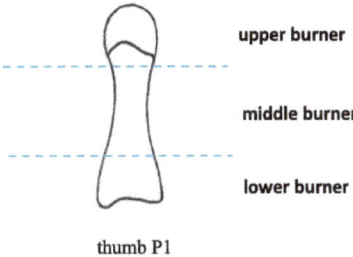

→ Pubic bone (dermis).

→ Inferior side of the chin (surface).

To differentiate resonance and circulation blockages:
→ Inguinal fold (palm/surface) = resonance.
→ Lower extremity of the sternum (palm/surface) = circulation.

Notes:

→ We can also find out the location of the resonance blockage on the Ren Mai through interrogating the palmaris longus tendon at the proximal level of the wrist.

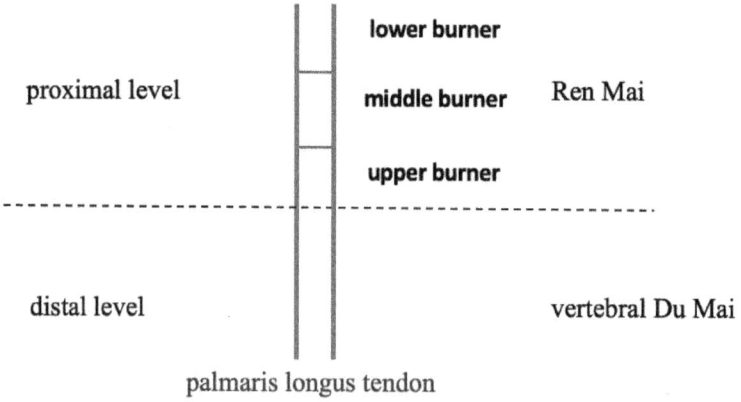

palmaris longus tendon

→ The anterior upper thigh centre is the same one for the Chong Mai. It does not include the circulation blockages of Ren Mai.
→ In case of Kidney-Yang (Yuan Qi) deficiency, one or more Ren Mai points at the Lower Burner level are often disturbed (resonance blockage).

II – CORRECTION

→ As for resonance blockages: One hand on the centre, the other one covers the Ren Mai until feeling the rope between both hands. The therapist, through the palpation of the first phalanx of the thumb and of the palmaris longus tendon, knows approximately in advance what area is affected on the Ren Mai.
→ As for circulation blockages: The practitioner lets one hand glide along the Ren Mai until he feels an obstacle that keeps his hand from gliding. He strokes this area a couple of times until the bumping sensation disappears.

DU MAI (central reservoir of Yang energies)

The Fire of Ming Men (Yuan Qi, Kidney-yang) provides heat for all the body (it is the Root of the Yang energy). It is concentrating at the DM 4 point.

The Du Mai has been studied in chapter VIII, "The emotional chains of Du Mai, Stomach and Gall Bladder channels".

CHONG MAI "the Sea of the 5 organs and 6 viscera" (Ling Shu)

Also called "the Sea of the 12 channels" and "the Sea of Blood".

The Chong Mai is related to the Kidneys, to Yuan and Jing Qi.

At the ST 30, the Chong Mai entry and starter point, the energies manufactured by the 3 burners are "spiritualized" by the Shen energy descending through Xu Li. This point is utilized when the energies remain blocked in the burners.

The Chong Mai points from KD 11 to KD 21, called by J. Pialoux "function Front-Mu points", control the distribution of energies to the organs and viscera.

Distribution order is the following:

ST 30	➡	(PC)
KD 11	➡	HT
KD 12	➡	SI
KD 13	➡	UB
KD 14	➡	LU
KD 15	➡	LI
KD 16	➡	KD
KD 17	➡	ST
KD 18	➡	SP
KD 19	➡	TW
KD 20	➡	GB
KD 21	➡	LV

I – OVERALL CONTROL

➔ Centre: anterior upper thigh (surface). This centre is the same one for the Ren Mai
➔ First metacarpal's head (osseous)
➔ Inguinal fold (dermis)
➔ Anterior upper thigh (palm/surface)

→ Dorsal side of the first metacarpal's base (surface)

II - DERTERMINING THE DISTURBED ENERGETIC FUNCTION

It is done through an osseous interrogation of the radius, at the proximal level of the wrist. This test is the same one for the Jing Bie Front-Mu points.

III - CORRECTION

One hand on the centre, the other one searching for the rope on the related Chong Mai point

DAI MAI

I - OVERALL CONTROL

→ Centre: greater trochanter (surface)
→ First metacarpal's neck (osseous)
→ Lateral extremity of the inguinal fold (dermis)
→ Top of the iliac crest, on the lateral side of the trunk (palm/surface)

II - CORRECTION

One hand on the centre, the other one looks for the rope on the GB 26, GB 27 or GB 28 points.

Note:

→ Often blocked in encystment problems and congestion of the pelvic region.

C - THE SECONDARY EXTRAORDINARY CHANNELS

The 4 Extraordinary Channels whose entry point is on the foot or the leg, drain off the energetic overload of the central coupled Extraordinary channels. If they fulfil their function, the area around their entry point is open. In order to test it, using the last phalanx of his three central fingers laid flat, the therapist palpates UB 62 (Yang Qiao Mai), KD 6 (Yin Qiao Mai), UB 63 (Yang Wei Mai), KD 9 (Yin Wei

Mai) areas and he questions vertically the surface (= epidermis) which responds or not (do not test just the point, allow a bit extra width).

I – OVERALL CONTROL

- → Umbilicus centre (surface)
- → Proximal half of the first metacarpal (osseous)
- → Posterior pelvis, lateral to the sacro-iliac articulations (palm/surface)
- → Greater wing of the sphenoid bone (temple) (dermis)

II – CORRECTION

The index finger of one hand placed horizontally on the related stripe of the umbilicus centre, the other hand looks for the rope, first on the entry point, then on the exit point and finally, on the others constituent points.

- → As for the Yang Wei Mai, the therapist first tests the UB 63 and GB 35, then the lower and posterior part of the skull. The higher the point, the stronger the disturbance in the Yang Wei Mai.
- → As for the Yin Wei Mai, first KD 9, then RM 22-23, finally the other constituent points.
- → As for the Yin Qiao Mai, first KD 6, then UB 1 and the other constituent point (KD 8).
- → As for the Yang Qiao Mai, first UB 62 then UB 1 and the other constituent points.

Notes:

- → Frequent blockages of the Yang Wei Mai in resonance with the thyroid gland, causing hypo or hyperthyroidism, nodules and with the parathyroid glands leading particularly to muscle spasms (stiff neck, back pain, abdominal, laryngeal spasms). Many people suffering from thyroid disorders run out of time and they have to hurry all day long, which contributes to raise the fire of the Triple Warmer and aggravate the pathology. They must learn to manage their time.
- → Frequent blockages of the Yin Wei Mai, in relation to PC, resulting in anguish, precordalgia, tightness in throat or chest.
- → An imbalance of the Yang Qiao Mai can lead to insomnia.

D – THE MASTER POINTS

Each Extraordinary Channel is linked to one specific channel to which it distributes the energies. The master point acts as a faucet. For example, KD 6 point controls the passage from Yin Qiao Mai to the KD channel.

I – OVERALL CONTROL

- → Lower stripe of the umbilicus centre (surface).
- → Acromio-clavicle articulation (surface).
- → Lateral side of the 5th metatarsal head (dermis).
- → Lateral extremity of the pelvis posterior side (palm/surface).

II – DETERMINING THE AFFECTED MASTER POINT

Through the osseous interrogation of the finger interphalangeal articulations (except for the thumb).
See plate 24 « Decoding of the Extraordinary Channels on the hand ».

III – CORRECTION

The index finger of one hand placed horizontally on the lower stripe of the umbilicus centre, the other hand on the master point.

E – THE CEPHALIC PSYCHO-SOMATIC GENERATOR = GB 1 TO GB 9 POINTS

These are the control and regulation points of the Extraordinary Channels, located on and around the greater wing of the sphenoid bone, at the centre of the head from a side view.
Decoding of GB 1 to GB 9 (Ben Shen is currently referred to as GB 13 by the Peking academy) points:

GB 1	➡	liaison Ren Mai-Du Mai
GB 2	➡	Yin Wei Mai
GB 3	➡	Yin Qiao Mai
GB 4	➡	Yang Wei Mai
GB 5	➡	Chong Mai

GB 6 → Dai Mai
GB 7 → Yang Qiao Mai
GB 8 → Du Mai
GB 9 → Ren Mai
(actual GB 13)

We shall also study the relationship of these points to the Heart channel (see chapter XII: « The specific centre of the Heart channel »).

I – OVERALL CONTROL

→ Sternoclavicular articulation (surface).
→ Lateral side of the knee (dermis).
→ Greater trochanter (palm/surface).
→ The centre is the vertex (with the emotional chains).

II – DETERMINING THE AFFECTED EXTRAORDINARY CHANNEL

It is done through a vertical osseous interrogation of the head and base of the four finger metacarpal bones (concerning the thumb, see chapter XXVII « the 3 Dan Tian »). The decoding of the Extraordinary Channels on the hand is illustrated on plate 24. If the head and base of the 5th metacarpal bone are blocked, the related point is GB 1.

III – CORRECTION

One hand on the GB cranial point related to the Extraordinary Channel, the other one looks for the rope on the vertex centre.

Note:

→ Frequent blockages of Yang Wei Mai and Yin Wei Mai (GB 4 and GB 2 are the related points).

F – MUSCLE DECODING

The thigh adductor muscles are in resonance with the Extraordinary Channels and give a general indication about their disturbance.

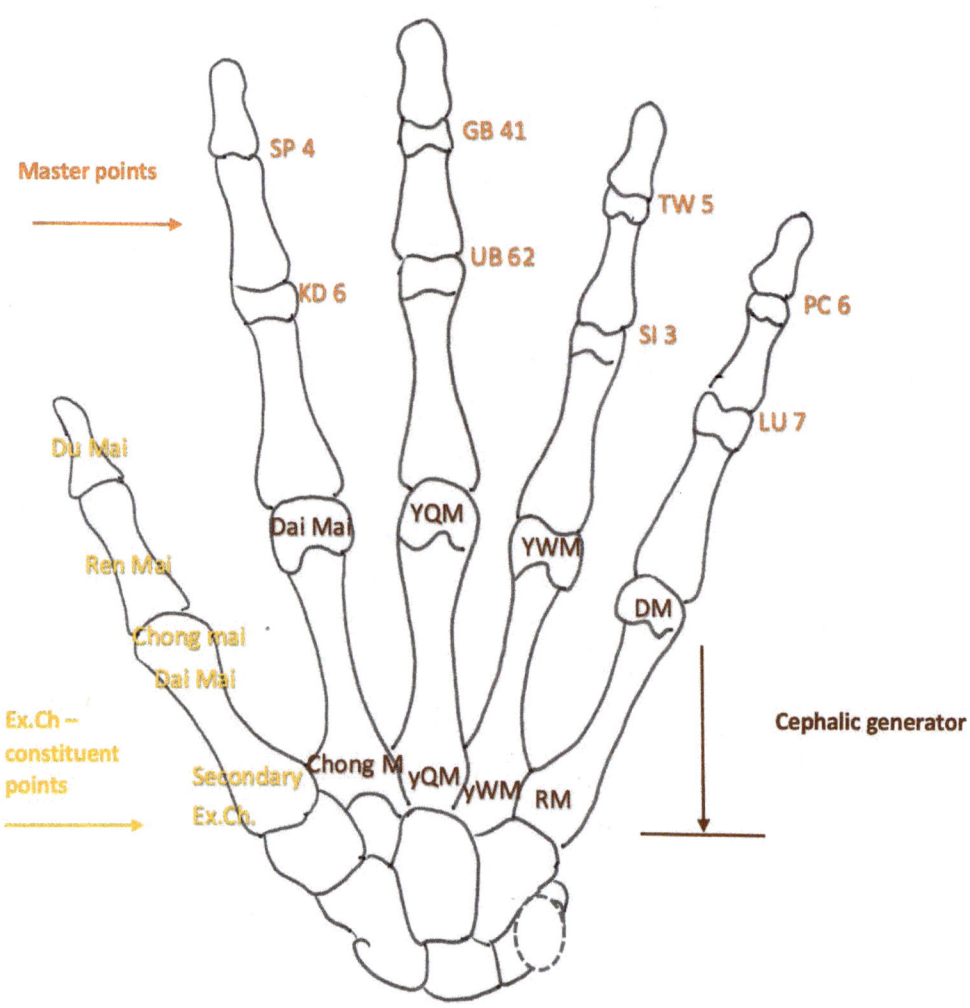

PLATE 24: THE EXTRAORDINARY CHANNELS ON THE HAND DORSAL SIDE (OSSEOUS)

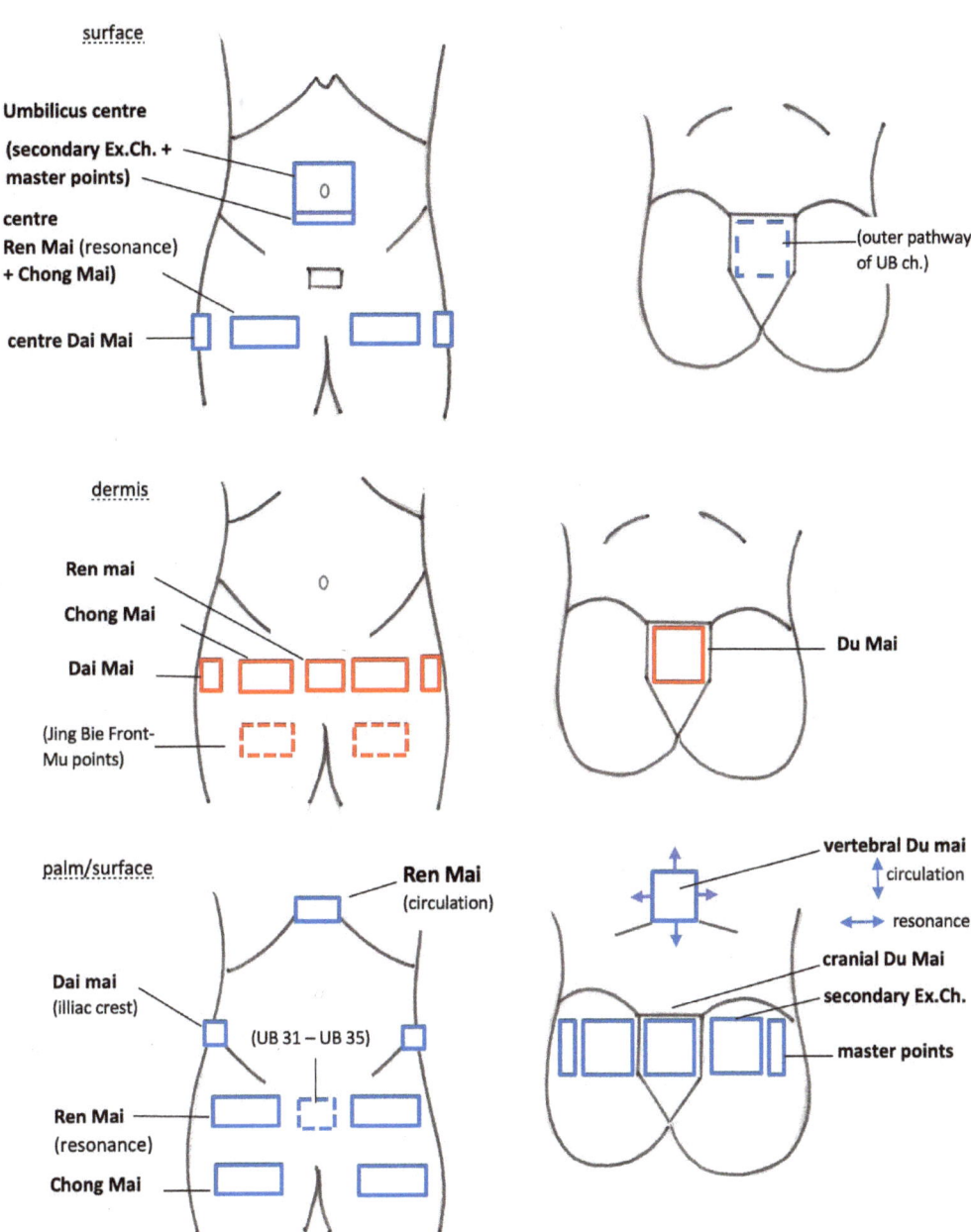

PLATE 25: THE EXTRAORDINARY CHANNELS ON THE PELVIS

X – THE SPECIFIC CENTRE OF THE GALL BLADDER CHANNEL

It is located on the lower cervical vertebrae (C6), related to the emotional level of the Gall Bladder. Qi stagnation in GB channel, caused by emotions (frustration, repressed anger, mental tension leading to headaches, muscle stiffness, neck and shoulder pain, lumbago, visceral spasms…), is often associated with a Yang Wei Mai disturbance (many points of Yang Wei Mai are GB channel points).

I – OVERALL CONTROL

Confirming the centre blockage:

- → Interphalangeal articulation of the great toe interrogated on the dorsal side (osseous).
- → Glabella (surface).
- → Lateral side of the shoulder (middle deltoid) (palm/surface, with a longitudinal impulse toward the feet).

II – CORRECTION

It is done with one hand on the centre, the other one looks for the rope on the GB channel, in its pathway along the fibula bone, since the therapist often finds it its lower half (GB 37- GB 38- GB 39). It allows to direct the energy down from the upper part of the body where most of symptoms are located (as the fire, caused by emotions, tends to go up).

X – THE SPECIFIC CENTRE OF THE GALL BLADDER CHANNEL

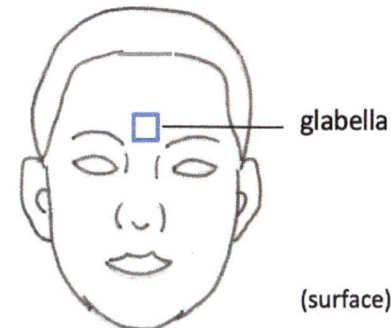

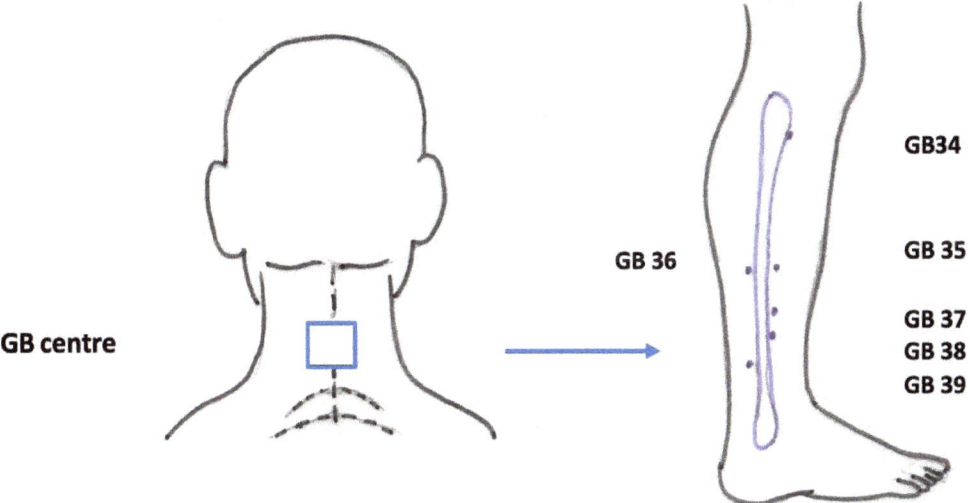

PLATE 26: THE SPECIFIC CENTRE OF THE GALL BLADDER CHANNEL

XI – THE SPECIFIC CENTRES OF THE SPLEEN

As all centres, they are both entry doors and correction areas.

A – CENTRE OF THE SPLEEN CHANNEL (SP 1 TO SP 11)

Located on the lateral side of the right costal margin (surface).
Confirming the centre blockage through the palpation of the lateral side of the left costal margin (palm/surface), at the level of the spleen organ itself.
This centre is related to 2 spleen functions:

I – BLOOD PRODUCTION

The control is done on the dorsal side of the first metatarsal head, with a crosswise osseous palpation (the therapist tests both sides because the centre does not indicate which one is affected) or on the medial side of the knees (surface).
The correction is made with one hand on the centre, the other one searches for the rope while palpating the points of the spleen channel (SP 1 to SP 11), starting particularly with SP 6 and SP 10 which are major blood points (often blocked in case of Blood and Yin deficiencies).

II – IMMUNE DEFENCE

(The spleen – thymus system is involved in immune deficiencies, pathologies as flu, mononucleosis…)
The control is done on the medial side of the first metatarsal head on both sides with a dermis palpation or on the sternum manubrium with a surface palpation.
The correction is made with one hand on the centre, the other one looks for the rope on the SP 1 to SP 11 points (SP 3 and SP 10 are the most frequent ones).

B – CENTRE OF THE SPLEEN CHAIN

Located on the anterior mid-thigh.
The chain of the spleen channel (from SP 12 to SP 21) is related to the 6 phases of disease described in chapter IV.
Confirmation of the centre blockage through palpation at the same level (anterior mid-thigh), with the hand palm, lengthways (toward the feet or the head).
The spleen chain decoding follows the order of the function Back- Shu points:

SP 21 ➡ KD

XI – THE SPECIFIC CENTRES OF THE SPLEEN

SP 20	➡	LU
SP 19	➡	LV
SP 18	➡	HT
SP 17	➡	SP
SP 16	➡	ST
SP 15	➡	LI
SP 14	➡	SI
SP 13	➡	UB
SP 12	➡	GB

I – SPECIFIC CONTROL

At the sternum level:

→ Manubrium (dermis), as for the Yang phases of disease (I-II-III).
→ Sternal angle, junction between the manubrium and the sternum body (dermis), as for the Yin phases (IV-V-VI).

At the foot level:

→ Scaphoid tubercle (surface), as for the Yang phases.
→ Medial side of the first metatarsal base (surface), as for the Yin phases.

II – DETERMINING THE DISTURBED ENERGETIC FUNCTION

It is done through a surface interrogation of the central groove (medial to the palmaris longus tendon) at the proximal level of the wrist.

→ Concerning the Yang phases, the blocked Element position indicates the Yang channel (Tai Yang, Yang Ming or Shao Yang) and therefore the related Yang phase (I-II-III).

Example:

→ If the Metal position is blocked, the patient presents then an inflammatory phase (phase II related to LI – ST).
A blocked Earth position also indicates an inflammatory phase; in this case, the SP 16 point (ST point) will be corrected in relation to the centre. In order to determine the body region affected by this inflammatory phase (it might be any organ or viscera, an articulation, a tooth…), the therapist puts down lightly the fingertips of one hand along the dorsal side of the 3rd metacarpal bone as the other one strokes the surface of the body. The same goes for the other Yang phases.
→ Concerning the Yin phases, the blocked position on the wrist indicates the disturbed energetic function, either the organ or the viscera can be affected (for instance, the Large Intestine can be found on the Yin phases). The therapist may confirm this with one hand on the dorsal side of 3rd

metatarsal bone, the other one stroking the trunk surface.
Confirmation through the palpation of the related points.

III – CORRECTION

It is done with one hand on the centre, the other one on the spleen chain point related to the blocked position on the wrist. In case of blockage on the Fire Minister position, the therapist takes **as for TW, the TW 15 – GB 21 points and as for PC, ST 10 point** which seems to be the counterpart of C7, a "PC vertebra", at the front of the body.

To sum up:

→ Any organ or viscera may be found on one of the 6 phases of disease. The spleen chain allows for a specific correction.
→ In the Yang phases, the centre is corrected in relation to the point corresponding to the viscera whose position on the wrist is blocked.
→ In the Yin phases, the centre is corrected in relation to the point corresponding to the organ or to the viscera whose position on the wrist is blocked.

Notes:

A few clarifications about the Fire Minister whose related points are not on the spleen channel (TW 15 - GB 21 and ST 10):

→ As for TW, from the 3rd metacarpal (Yang phases) or the 3rd metatarsal (Yin phases), the practitioner often finds a blocked area on the anterior side of the neck, at the thyroid and parathyroid glands level, TW being related to the Yang Wei Mai whose master point is TW 5.
→ As for PC, from the 3rd metatarsal (Yin phases), the practitioner finds:
  → either a zone in the cardiac region which indicates cardiovascular problems, in relation to phase IV and especially phase V (high blood pressure, coronary problems, stroke, arteritis…).
  → Or, in relation to the phase VI of neoplasm, a body region which is linked to it.

  This blockage seldom appears in the beginning of the disease. Besides, it is not constant. Its correction does not claim to have an influence on the tumoral process but can remove an energy stagnation in the affected area- a heavy and dense zone to palpate (that the therapist finds from the 3rd metatarsal) - and strengthen the energy of the disturbed organ.

XI – THE SPECIFIC CENTRES OF THE SPLEEN

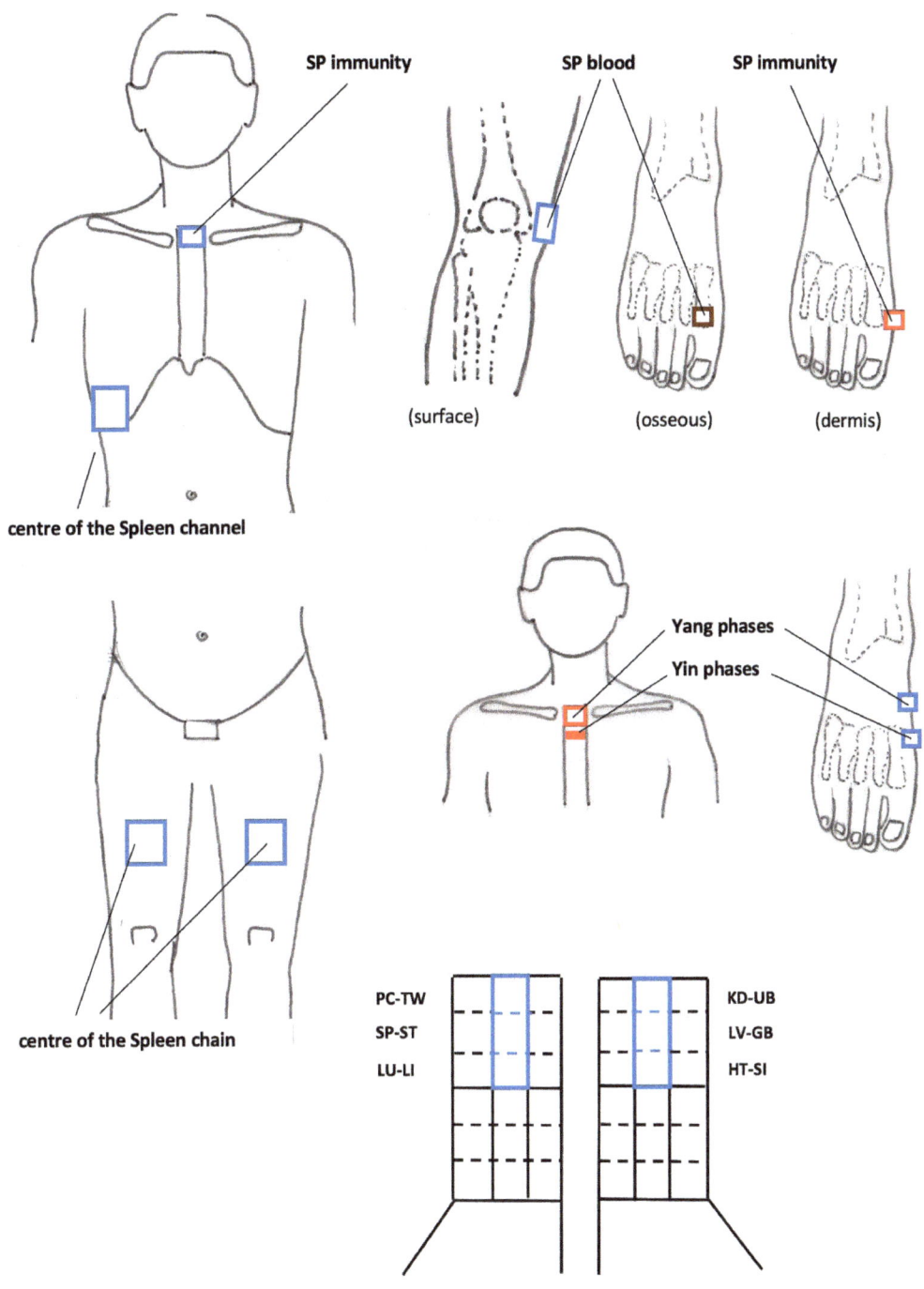

PLATE 27: THE SPECIFIC CENTRE OF THE GALL BLADDER CHANNEL

XII – THE SPECIFIC CENTRE OF THE HEART CHANNEL

Located in the upper third of the sternum body, below the manubrium.
The Heart houses the Shen (the Mind) and can be affected by all extreme emotions.
This centre is often blocked in depressive states and cases of emotional loss.

I – OVERALL CONTROL

- → Centre: upper third of the sternum body (surface).

Confirmation du blocage du centre:

- → Inferior side of the floor of mouth (dermis).
- → Vertebral region T4-T6 (palm/surface with an upward impulse).

II – DETERMINING THE DISTURBED POINT OF THE HEART CHANNEL

It is done through the palpation of the dermis, in the ulnar groove, at the distal level of the wrist.

Example:

- → If the Wood position is blocked, HT 9 (Wood point of the heart channel) is closed on the side of the blocked sternum hemi-centre.

III – CORRECTION

It is done in 2 steps:

- → 1st step: one hand on the Heart channel point, the other one examines the points from GB 1 to GB 9- actual GB 13- in order to find the rope. After it loosens up, the Heart point starts opening (GB/HT axis on the spiritual plane).
- → 2nd step: the therapist keeps one hand on the Heart channel point and looks for the rope on the centre, on the sternum, which allows to open the point completely.

XII – THE SPECIFIC CENTRE OF THE HEART CHANNEL

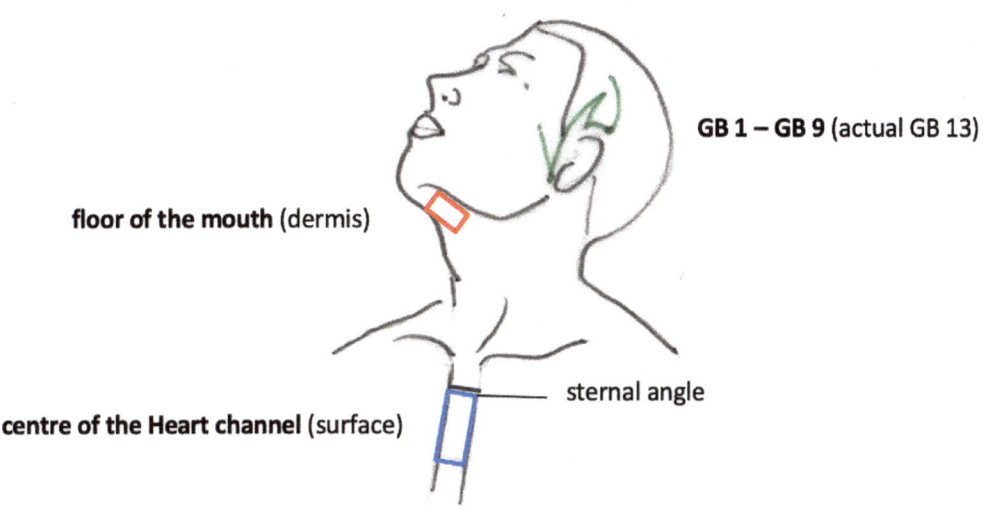

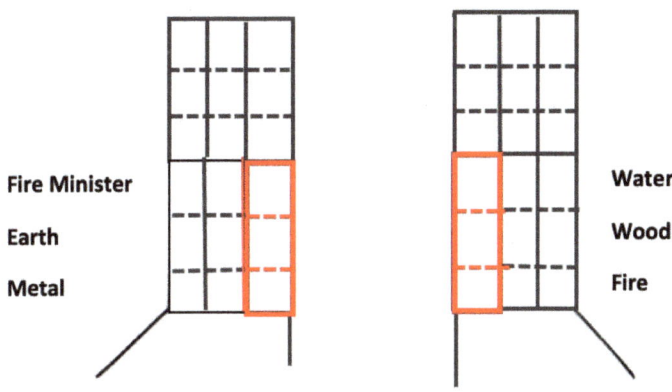

PLATE 28: SPECIFIC CENTRE OF THE HEART CHANNEL

XIII – THE OCCIPITAL CENTRE

Related to:
→ The outer pathway of the UB channel.
→ The UB 31 to UB 35 points, on the sacrum.

The centre is located on the skull base and its palpation is done with 4 fingers placed crosswise, 2 fingers on the occiput, the 2 others on C1 and C2.

A – THE OUTER PATHWAY OF THE URINARY BLADDER CHANNEL

It is related to the spiritual plane and to the "Five Shen" (Shen, Hun, Po, Yi and Zhi). Associated with the notion of Kouei (Gui) whose ideogram is contained with the one of the Po and the Hun. Referring to modern research in psychology, we can mention the psychogenealogical approach related to Ancestral Memory[1] and Grof's perinatal matrices[2] which correspond to the four distinct stages in birth and the trauma associated with each stage.

Decoding is as follows:

UB 42	(T3)	→	LU
UB 43	(T4)	→	LI
UB 44	(T5)	→	HT
UB 45	(T6)	→	SI
UB 46	(T7)	→	UB
UB 47	(T9)	→	LV
UB 48	(T10)	→	GB
UB 49	(T11)	→	SP
UB 50	(T12)	→	ST
UB 51	(L1)	→	TW
UB 52	(L2)	→	KD
UB 53	(S2)	→	PC

I – OVERALL CONTROL

→ Sacrum (surface) with the 4 fingers placed crosswise.
→ Lateral side of the ankle (dermis), with 1 finger crosswise on the lower extremity of the lateral malleolus, a second finger just below on the lateral side of the calcaneum.
→ Clavicle (palm/surface).

---

1. Schutzenberger Anne Ancelin, "The Ancestor syndrome: Transgenerational Psychotherapy and the Hidden Links in the Family Tree", Routledge Publisher
2. Grof Stanislav, "Realms of the Human Unconscious", Souvenir Press Ltd

II – DETERMINING THE DISTURBED ENERGETIC FUNCTION

It is done with a surface interrogation of the ulnar groove at the proximal level of the wrist.

Confirmation through a vertical palpation of the metatarsal bones, at the osseous level:

Foot M1	➡	Earth
M2	➡	Metal
M3	➡	Water
M4	➡	Wood
M5	➡	Fire – Fire Minister

III – CORRECTION

It is done with one hand on the occipital centre, the other one on the related point of the outer pathway of UB channel.

Notes:
→ The observation shows frequent blockages among agitated or anguished infants and young children, also in the case of enuresis.
→ Emotional shocks, anniversary of a traumatic event in the family history (Anniversary Syndrome) can reactivate blockages in the outer pathway of the UB channel.

B – UB 31 TO UB 35 POINTS

Related to the energy movement that animates the sacrum, called Primary Respiratory Movement in osteopathy, which must be differentiated from the articular mobility of the sacrum in relation to the iliac bone and the 5th lumbar vertebra.

I – OVERALL CONTROL

→ Lateral side of the 5th metatarsal head (surface).
→ T4-T5 vertebral region, near the spinous process (dermis).
→ Pubic bone (palm/surface).

II – CORRECTION

It is done with one hand on the occipital centre, the other one looks for the rope on the sacrum, at the level of the UB 31 to UB 35 points.

Note:
→ Frequent blockages in lower back pain, mainly in the sacrum area, and sciatica. Repercussion all over the vertebral column.

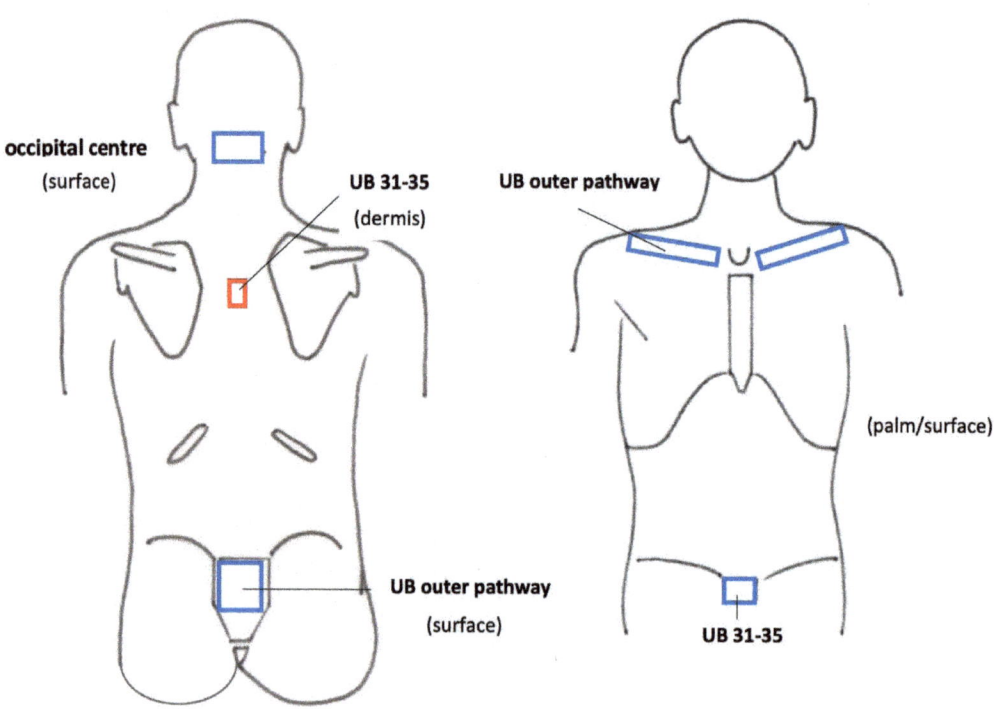

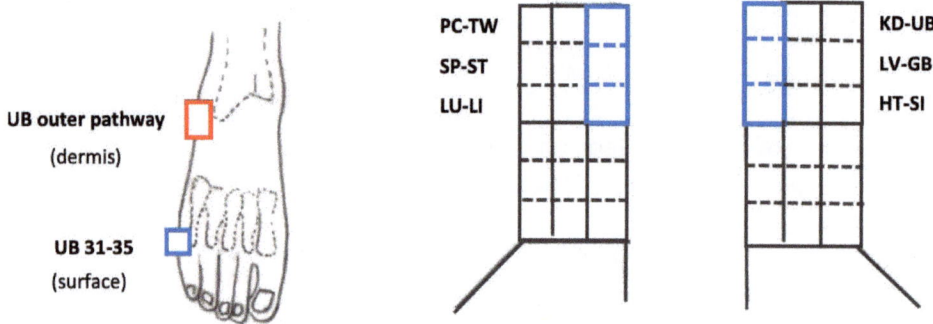

PLATE 29: THE OCCIPITAL CENTRE

XIV – THE FRONTAL CENTRE

Located on the hairline, at the level of the DM 24 area and related to the head points of the Yang channels.

Confirmation of the centre blockage through a dermis palpation of the dorsal side of the great toe's 2nd phalanx, below the nail.

I – DETERMINING THE AFFECTED CHANNEL

It is done on the side of the blocked hemi-centre and great toe:

→ Through a crosswise osseous palpation on the hand metacarpals, the therapist covering up all the metacarpal bone with his fingers:

    M2 ➡ GB
    M3 ➡ UB
    M4 ➡ SI-TW
    M5 ➡ ST-LI

→ Through a surface hand palm interrogation lengthways, toward the feet (the sensation under the hand is stronger downwards than upwards) at the level of:

    The temple (great wing of the sphenoid) ➡ GB
    The area just behind the temple ➡ SI-TW
    The cheek (maxilla) ➡ ST-LI
    The forehead, on the central line ➡ UB

II – CORRECTION

It is done with one hand on the blocked frontal half centre, the other one looks for the rope while palpating the different points of the affected channel on the same side (as for as the GB and UB channels are concerned, start with the face points).

Note:
→ The cephalic GB points related to the emotional GB chain and the cephalic generator or the Heart channel are not included in this control.

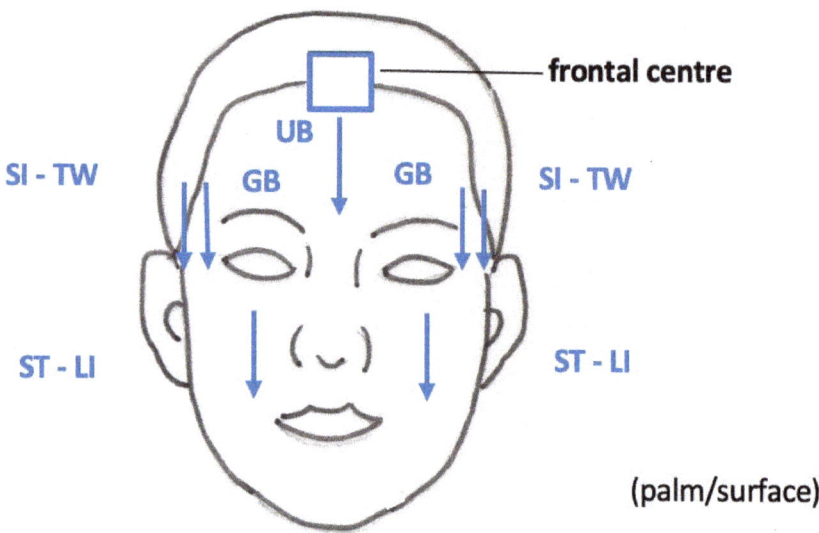

PLATE 30: THE FRONTAL CENTRE

XV – THE PHYSICAL TRAUMA

A – THE TRAUMATIC BLOCKAGES

Joint and muscle blockages (i.e. a restriction in their mobility) caused by falls, blows or improper movements, are corrected from the centre of the ankle.

I – OVERALL CONTROL

The therapist interrogates the surface all around the ankle with one finger placed crosswise on the extremity of the malleoli, the other one just below.

II – CORRECTION

The practitioner keeps one hand down on the blocked area of the ankle, the other one goes down along the lateral side of the body, on the surface, looking for the rope. This second hand does not indicate the location of the traumatic blockage but its height in the body. The corrections are always made on this lateral line (vertebral disorders included), which goes from the vertex to the 5th toe and from the acromion to the thumb - note that the therapist does not need to know the precise location of the traumatic blockage in order to correct it (it could be found, through an osseous or muscle vertical interrogation, in the horizontal stripe going through the correction area on the lateral side of the body).

For the same trauma, several areas in the centre are usually affected because different muscles and ligaments are involved, that is why it is necessary to interrogate all around the ankle as well as the Achilles tendon.

Notes:

→ All articular blockages (vertebral or peripheral) have 2 possible aetiologies:
  → A trauma: they are treated then from the centre of the ankle.
  → A disturbance in the energetic system (for instance, a blockage of the fibula bone caused by a stagnation in the GB channel or a T9 blockage by a stagnation in the Liver): they are then treated from the other controls of the reading grid.

→ The T4 - T5 vertebral area, which is the mechanical centre of the vertebral column, allows to verify the mechanical equilibrium of the body.
  The therapist lays his fingers flat lengthways on the T4 - T5 area and interrogates the surface (epidermis) with an impulse directed upwards. (Its blockage in all directions means that the therapist cannot interpret it as previously mentioned).
  If this area is free, the therapist will not find any traumatic blockage at the level of the vertebral column and lower limbs nor a disturbance of the occiput and sacrum energy movements, and vice versa.
  Similarly to what is done for the centres seated on the midline, he can interrogate one half of the area to determine the side of the blockage.

→ If the T4 – T5 blockage persists after treatment, the therapist must be steered towards a problem of foot supports or visual asymmetry as well as bad dental occlusion – in this last case, he may confirm it through a vertical osseous palpation of the first phalanx of the 3rd finger, in resonance with the mandible, or of the temporomandibular joint, in the GB 2 area.
  Referring the patient to a specialized therapist in these fields might prove to be necessary.

The T4 – T5 control will allow to verify afterwards the accuracy of the corrections that were made.

→ The traumatic centre of the ankle does not include the energy movements of the sacrum and the occiput. These are treated with the UB 31 to UB 35 points (see chapter XIII: The occipital centre) and the « Window of the Sky points » (see chapter XVII).

→ In neck pains, the diaphragm is often affected because of its relation to C3 - C4 - C5. Its correction is made on the lateral and lower side of the thoracic cage from the blocked area on the ankle.

B - TENDINITIS

Tendinitis caused by mechanical over-exertion are treated from GB 34 which is the converging point of sinews.

I - OVERALL CONTROL

→ Dorsal side of the 5th metatarsal base (surface)
→ Below the tubercle of the chin, lateral to the symphysis (dermis).
→ Anterior mid-thigh (palm/surface).

Note:

→ In case of a blockage, the GB 34 point is closed and the tissue below the head of the fibula is often hard or tense.

II - CORRECTION

It is done with a deep, strong palpation, with the fingertips, one hand on GB 34, the other looks for the rope(s) on the painful area indicated by the patient (repeat the correction if the blockage reappears during the treatment).

XV – THE PHYSICAL TRAUMA

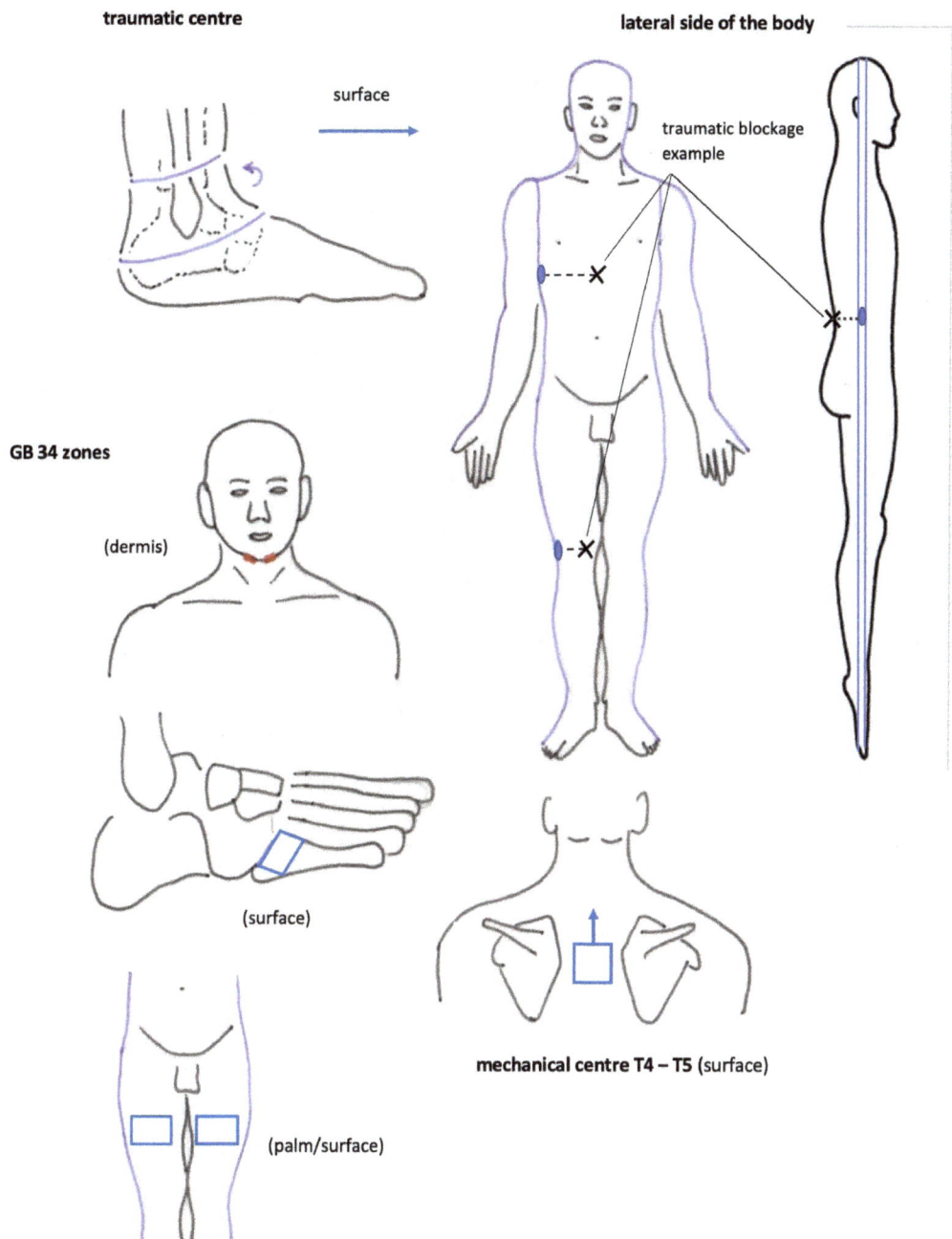

PLATE 31: THE PHYSICAL TRAUMA

XVI – THE BARRIERS

The organism can protect itself in case of heavy stress, physical or psychological, by putting up a barrier on a weakened organ. Useful at first, this protection, if it remains in place afterwards, may create an energetic disturbance, manifested particularly, in the course of a treatment, by a relapse after a short improvement period.

List of the « barrier » (guan) points of the organs:

- LI ➡ DM 3 (YaoYang guan)
- KD ➡ KD 18 (Shiguan)
- UB ➡ UB 46 (Geguan)
- SI ➡ RM 4 (Guan Yuan)
- LV ➡ LV 7 (Xiguan)
- GB ➡ GB 33 (Yng guan)
- SP ➡ ST 31 (Biguan)
- ST ➡ ST 22 (Guanmen)
- PC ➡ PC 6 (Neiguan)
- TW ➡ TW 5 (Waiguan)
- LU ➡ TW 1 (Guanchong)
- HT ➡ no barrier point

I – OVERALL CONTROL

The "barrier" centre is located at the level of the acromion (lateral side of the shoulder). The interrogation is on the surface as for all centres.

Confirmation through the dermis palpation of the glabella (Yin Tang point area) and through the palm/surface palpation of the supraspinatus fossa of the scapula, with an upward impulse.

II – DETERMINING THE AFFECTED ENERGETIC FUNCTION

It is done by interrogating the surface (epidermis) of the dorsal side of the wrist, at the distal level, between the two bones of the forearm, with the usual localization of the Element positions.

Confirmation through the palpation of the related « barrier » point, on the blocked side in the overall control.

III – CORRECTION

It is done with one hand on the « barrier » point, the other one on the centre (acromion).

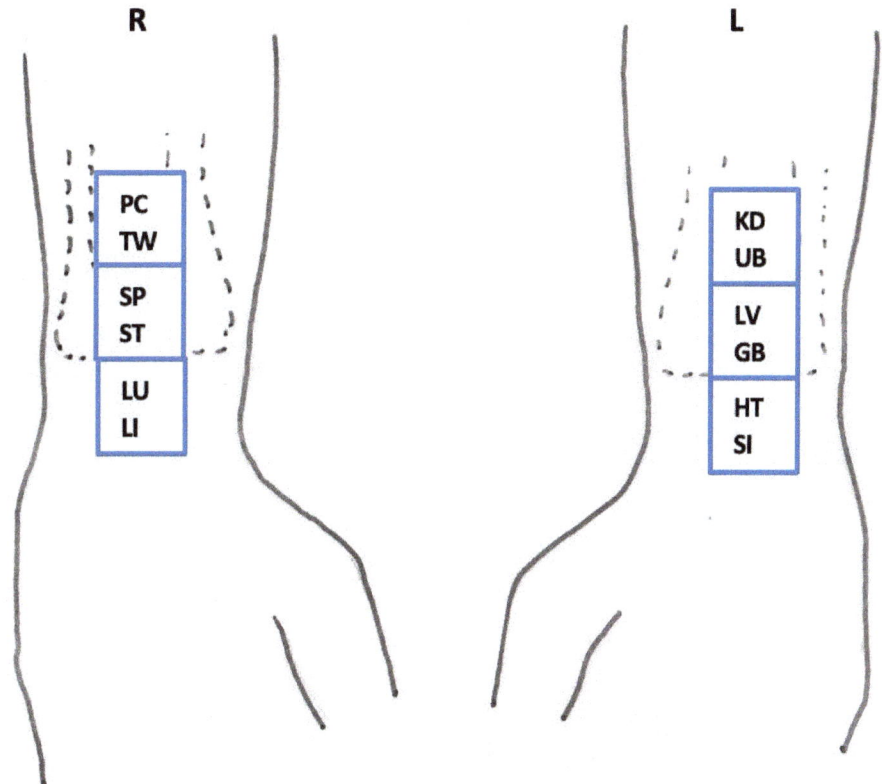

PLATE 32: LOCATION OF THE ENERGETIC FUNCTIONS AT THE DORSAL SIDE OF THE WRIST

COMPLEMENTARY CONTROLS

- → XVII   The Window of the Sky Points
- → XVIII   The Pathway of Liquids
- → XIX   Stomach Chain and Energy Stagnation
- → XX   The Pericardium Channel
- → XXI   Chain from KD 22 to KD 27
- → XXII   The General Functions
- → XXIII   The Luo Points of the 12 Channels
- → XXIV   Circulation Blockages in the 12 Channels
- → XXV   The Tendino-muscular Channels
- → XXVI   Elimination Function of ST 36, ST 37, ST 39 Points
- → XXVII   The 3 Dan Tian

XVII – THE WINDOW OF THE SKY POINTS

The basic function of this group of points is to facilitate the flow of energy between the head and the rest of the body, the Heaven and Earth of the human being. An entry door for external disturbing energies, particularly the Wind (Feng), they also constitute a safety lock to keep them from penetrating in depth. Emotional tensions may as well close down the Window of the Sky points resulting in excess energy in the head (headaches, conjunctivitis …) or cervical blockages.

The list of these points is variable according to the authors. The most mentioned are: ST 9 - LI 18 – SI 16 – TW 16 – UB 10 – GB 20 (named Fengchi and constituent point of Yang Wei Mai and Yang Qiao Mai) – and we add DM 16 (named Fengfu and constituent point of Yang Wei Mai).

In practice, we consider 2 horizontal stripes:
→ A superior one, at the base of the skull (occiput-C1-C2), going from DM 16 to the mastoid apophysis.
→ An inferior one, including ST 9, LI 18, SI 16 practically lined up.

I – OVERALL CONTROL

→ Mid-transverse crease of the wrist (dermis)
→ Sternum manubrium (palm/surface) with:
    → Horizontal interrogation ↔ for the superior stripe.
    → Longitudinal interrogation ↕ for the inferior stripe.

II – CORRECTION

→ As for the superior stripe, two steps:
    → 1ˢᵗ step: one hand is searching, through a vertical osseous palpation, with fingertips, for an area which does not respond, on the lateral part of the sternal angle (junction between the manubrium and the body of the sternum).
    → 2ⁿᵈ step: the therapist keeps one hand on this area, the other hand's fingers with a deep palpation, on the occiput-C1-C2, covers all the superior stripe from DM 16 to the mastoid apophysis, searching for one or several ropes.

→ As for the inferior stripe, two steps:
  → 1st step: one hand is searching through a vertical osseous palpation, with fingertips, for an area which does not respond on the medial part of the sternal angle.
  → 2nd step: the therapist keeps one hand down on this area, the other one covers all the inferior stripe.

Remarques:

→ The blockage of the Window of the Sky points in the superior stripe disturbs the occipital energy movement (called Primary Respiratory Movement in osteopathy), that we must differentiate from the articular blockage between the occiput (C0 in osteopathy) and C1.
Confirmation through a vertical osseous palpation of the thumb's first phalanx which is in resonance with the occiput.
→ In case of direct shocks on the head or of whiplash, the articular blockages of occiput-C1 and other vertebrae are corrected from the centre of the ankle, while the blockage of the occiput energy movement is corrected from the Window of the Sky points.

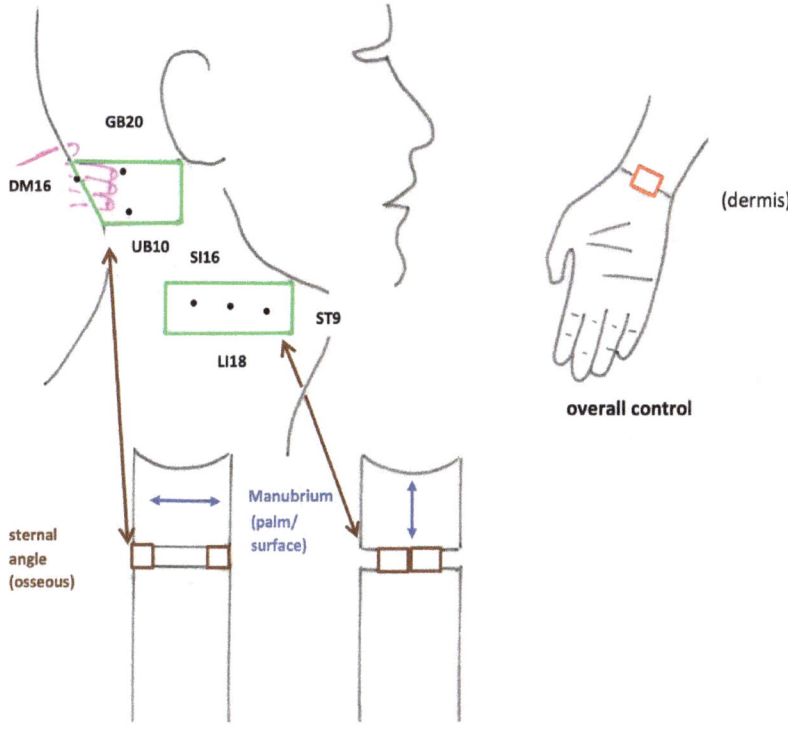

PLATE 33: THE WINDOW OF THE SKY POINTS
XVIII – THE PATHWAY OF LIQUIDS

A – THE TRIPLE WARMER

The Triple Warmer has an irrigating function; it regulates the circulation of water (fluids) throughout the body. It helps the spleen to drain dampness. We study this aspect of the Triple Warmer in this chapter (the other aspect is the « Pathway of Fire » related to the Fire Minister and Yuan Qi).

I – OVERALL CONTROL

- → Dorsal side of the 3rd metatarsal base (dermis).
- → Dorsal side of the wrist (surface).
- → 12th rib (palm/surface).

The Triple Warmer channel on the same side is blocked when it is palpated.

II – CORRECTION

The therapist looks for the TW point which does not respond (TW 1, TW 2 or TW 3 are often closed).
He keeps one hand down on this point and, with the other one, looks for the rope in an area located slightly above and to the left of the umbilicus, corresponding anatomically to the cisterna chyli.

Notes:

- → The cisterna chyli is a dilated sac which receives the lymphatic drainage in the abdomen. It is formed by the junction of lumbar and intestinal lymphatic trunks, continues as the thoracic duct which empties into the left subclavian vein.
- → This function of the TW is often disturbed in all lymphatic circulatory disorders, venous insufficiency manifested by heaviness in the legs, oedema of lower or upper limbs...

B – THE SP 6 POINT

We include in this chapter the SP 6 point in its drainage function particularly of the lower burner (elimination of Damp-Heat and Dampness - or of blood stagnation, which may cause pelvic congestion, haemorrhoids, circulatory problems of the lower limbs).

I – OVERALL CONTROL

- Lateral side of the 5th metatarsal base (dermis).
- Lower half of the patella (surface).
- 12th rib (palm/surface, with a longitudinal impulse, toward the head or the feet).

The SP 6 point is closed on the same side.

II – CORRECTION

It is done with one hand on the SP 6, the other one looks for the rope at the level of the lower burner, on the Spleen channel, from SP 12 to SP 15.

Notes:

- The blockage of the SP 6 point can be observed in localized blood stagnation, post-traumatic haematoma, for instance. Correction with one hand on SP 6 point, the other one looks for the rope at the level of the blood stagnation.
- The other organs which regulate the Pathway of Liquids are controlled in previous chapters.

XIX – STOMACH CHAIN AND ENERGY STAGNATION

The phase III of disease, of toxin deposit, is characterized by cyst formation, nodules, stones. In order to treat these energy stagnations, the Stomach must "digest" what it has covered with Earth at the organ level, in the three burners.

Reminder:

→ The Stomach chain (ST 11 to ST 30) at the emotional level has been studied in chapter VIII.

I – OVERALL CONTROL

→ Dorsal side of the interphalangeal articulation of the great toe (surface).
→ Anterior side of the chin (dermis).
→ Anterior side of the thoracic cage, below the pectoral region (palm/surface).

The GB 42 point is closed on the same side in case of blockage. It is the entry door to correct the energy stagnation from the Stomach chain.

II – DETERMINING THE LOCATION OF STAGNATION IN THE 3 BURNERS

→ The therapist questions the dermis of the central groove, at the proximal level of the wrist, on the blocked side in the overall control. The 3 positions are related to the 3 burners (upper burner -middle burner -lower burner from the distal to the proximal).

III – CORRECTION

→ It is done with one hand on the GB 42 point, the other one covers the portion of the Stomach chain on the same side, corresponding to the burner found on the wrist. After the loosening of the rope, the GB 42 point is open and the stagnation of the energy that the therapist could feel under his hand (a dense and heavy zone) disappears.

XIX – STOMACH CHAIN AND ENERGY STAGNATION

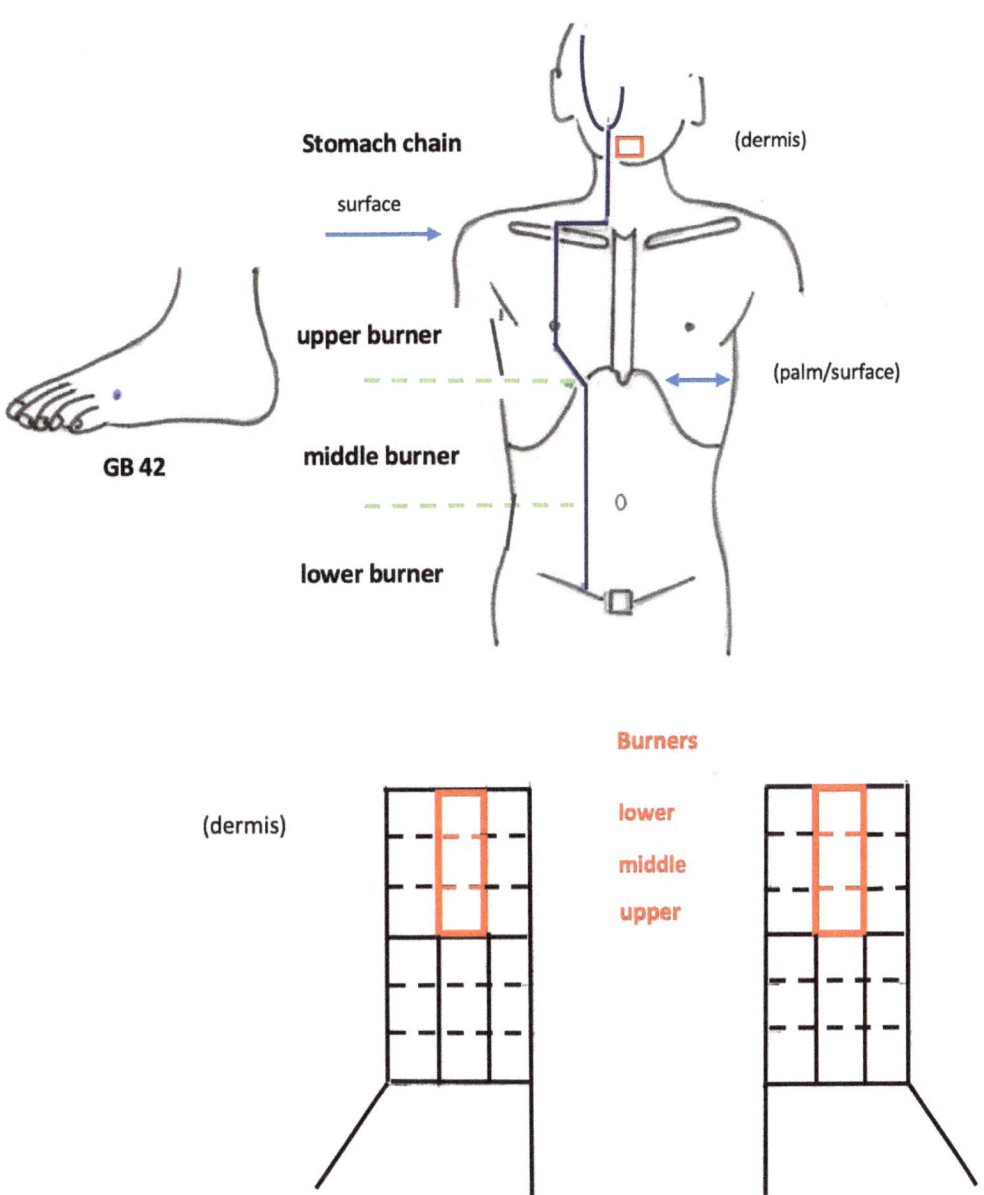

PLATE 34: STOMACH CHAIN AND ENERGY STAGNATION

XX – THE PERICARDIUM CHANNEL

The basic function of the Pericardium is to protect the Heart. It is this aspect, mainly on a physical level, that we consider in this chapter (even though the physical and emotional sides are intertwined). Its imbalance, resulting in chest or throat tightness and cardiovascular pathologies as high blood pressure, heart rate disorders, coronary problems, stroke, etc., can be improved by a specific correction of the PC channel.

(See also the Pericardium at the level of the Spleen chain related to the 6 phases of disease, in chapter XI).

Reminder:
The emotional aspect of the Pericardium has been studied with:
➔ The Yin Wei Mai whose master point is PC 6, in chapter IX
➔ The emotional chain of the Stomach channel in chapter VIII

I – OVERALL CONTROL

➔ Dorsal side of the great toe first phalanx (surface)
➔ Inferior extremity of the sternum (dermis)
➔ Anterior side of the thoracic cage, below the pectoral region (hand/palm with a longitudinal impulse)

II – DETERMINING THE DISTURBED POINT ON THE PERICARDIUM CHANNEL

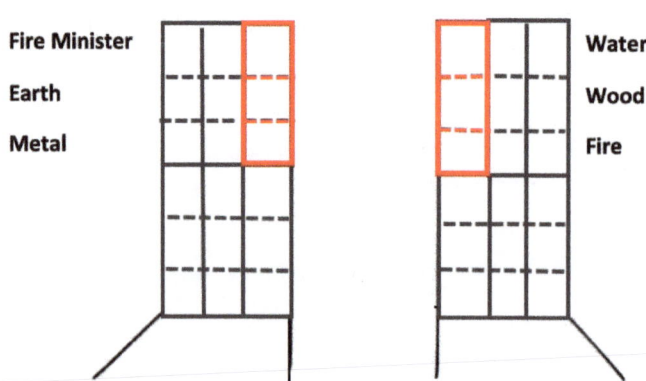

Example:

→ If the Water position is not free, the PC 3 (Water point of the PC channel) is closed on the blocked side in the overall control.

III – CORRECTION

→ The therapist puts one hand down on the PC point and, with the other one, he looks for the rope in the occipital area (anatomically at the level of the posterior part of the bulb and the nuclei of the vagus nerve (X); PC and TW are in resonance with the autonomic nervous system).

XXI – CHAIN FROM KD 22 TO KD 27

A deep emotional chain related to the Shen energy (the name of KD 23 is Shenfeng and the one of KD 25 is Shencang).

The correspondence to the 5 Elements is as follows:

KD 27	➡	Fire Minister
KD 26	➡	Water
KD 25	➡	Metal
KD 24	➡	Earth
KD 23	➡	Fire
KD 22	➡	Wood

I – OVERALL CONTROL

→ Dorsal side of the 2nd phalanx of the great toe (surface).
→ Upper third of the sternum body, below the manubrium (dermis).
→ T4-T5 vertebral area (palm/surface).

II – DETERMINING THE DISTURBED ENERGETIC FUNCTION

It is done through an osseous interrogation in the radial groove, at the distal level of the wrist (radius bone extremity).

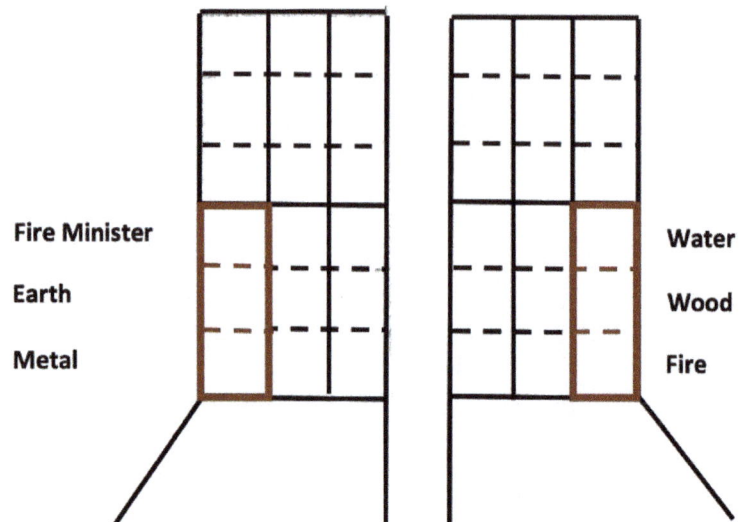

Confirmation through the palpation of the related point of the chain from KD 22 to KD 27 and of the related 5 Shu point of the KD channel.

Example:

➔ If the Water position on the wrist is blocked, KD 26 and KD 10 ("Water points") are closed on the blockage side in the overall control.

III – CORRECTION

Two steps:

➔ 1st step: one hand, through a vertical palpation with fingertips, searches on the sternum body for a blocked area at the osseous level, which does not respond (no osseous elasticity).

➔ 2nd step: the therapist keeps one hand on this area, the other one looks for the rope on the related point of the KD 22- KD 27 chain.

XXII – GENERAL FUNCTIONS

This study, which is made from major points of Energy, is focused on general functions.

- → "Liver" function: a draining function on the physical and emotional planes of which the LV 3 point is often utilized (and LV 10 – LV 11 – LV 12 specifically for the lower burner).

- → "Large Intestine" function: The Large Intestine is the organ of inflammation. LI 4 and LI 11 points allow to lower the fire in the organs.

- → "Earth" function: as a central Element, the Earth has a harmonizing and re-centring function. The major point is ST 36 which also allows to tonify Yang Energy.

A disturbance of these functions may affect each organ or viscera.

I – OVERALL CONTROL

- → Great trochanter (palm/surface, with a longitudinal impulse, toward the head or the feet).

II – SPECIFIC CONTROLS

- → Concerning the Earth function:
    - → Anterior part of the talus, between the malleoli (dermis)
    - → Superior half of the patella (surface)

- → Concerning the LV and LI functions:
    - → Pisiform (dermis)
    - → Medial side of the 1st metatarsal head (surface) ↗ LI 4, in the superior part
    ↘ LI 11, in the inferior part

→ Medial side of the 1st
→ metatarsal neck (surface)

LV 3, in the superior part
↗
↘
LV 10-11-12, in the inferior part

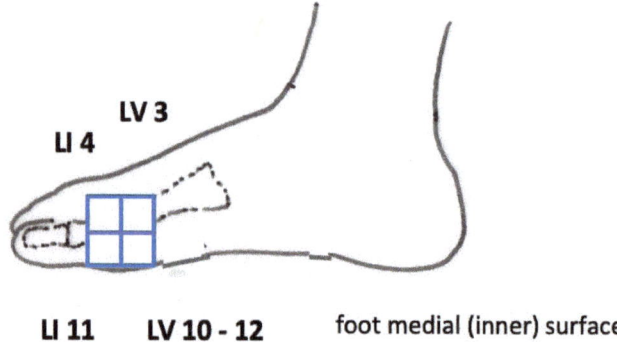

LI 4   LV 3

LI 11   LV 10 - 12   foot medial (inner) surface

III – DETERMINING THE DISTURBED ENERGETIC FUNCTION

It is done through a dermis interrogation of the central groove at the distal level of the wrist, medial to the palmaris longus tendon.

Note:
→ As for LV 10-11-12, the Water or Fire Minister position is blocked

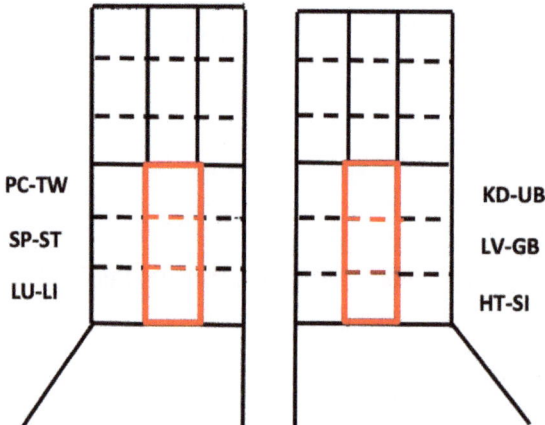

PC-TW   KD-UB
SP-ST   LV-GB
LU-LI   HT-SI

IV – CORRECTION

One hand on the major point, the other one covers the organ or viscera related to the blocked position on the wrist. As for LV 10-12 points, from the closed point on, the second hand looks for the rope at the level of the lower burner.

XXIII – THE LUO POINTS OF THE 12 CHANNELS

The Luo points open spaces in the body (most master points are Luo points). The transverse Luo channels connect the paired main channels (Yin and Yang) and, therefore, the organ (Zang) with the coupled viscera (Fu) which is also its emunctory. The organ Luo point is often combined with the Yuan-source point of the viscera in the treatments (mainly in this way to avoid the in-depth penetration of a disturbing energy into the organ).

Reminder:
→ List of Luo points: LI 6 - LU 7- UB 58 – KD 4 – GB 37 – LV 5 – SI 7 – HT 5 – ST 40 – SP 4 – TW 5 – PC 6

I - OVERALL CONTROL

→ The therapist puts his index finger down on the medial side of the 1st metatarsal bone, lengthwise; the impulse is on the surface, in the anterior/posterior axis of the foot
→ Dorsal side of the wrist (dermis)
→ Umbilical area (palm/surface with a longitudinal impulse, toward the head or the feet)

II - DETERMINING THE AFFECTED LUO POINT

The therapist questions the surface of the central groove, at the distal level of the wrist. Confirmation through the palpation of the Luo point of the related channels.

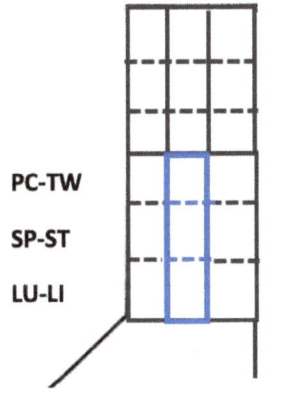
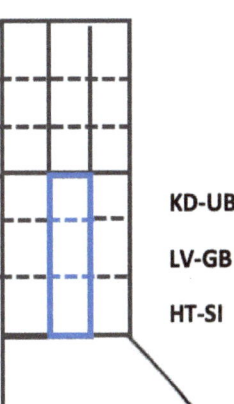

III – CORRECTION

- → Concerning the Luo point of the Yin channels (the most frequent case), one hand on the Luo point, the other one looks for the rope at the level of the coupled viscera or of the midday/midnight viscera in the horary cycle which is the second emunctory of an organ, or in the absence of rope on the viscera, on the organ itself. It allows to liberate an excess energy of an organ toward its emunctories.
- → Concerning the Luo point of the Yang channels, one hand on the Luo point, the second hand is on the related viscera.

Example:

- → As for the Luo point of the Lung channel (LU 7), the therapist looks for the rope on the large intestine or on the urinary bladder and, in the absence of rope on these two viscera, on the lung itself.

Notes:

- → As for TW, the therapist searches for an area near the front midline of the trunk.
- → The Great Luo of Stomach will be studied at the end of chapter XXV: *The tendino-muscular channels.*

XXIV – CIRCULATION BLOCKAGE IN THE 12 CHANNELS

It is the obstruction of the Energy flow on the pathway of a channel, mainly on the limbs, at the level of one point or between two points.

I – OVERALL CONTROL

- → The therapist puts his index finger down on the lateral side of the 5th metatarsal, lengthwise. The impulse is on the surface, in the anterior/posterior axis of the foot.
- → Dorsal side of the thumb's first phalanx (surface).
- → Umbilical area (palm/surface).

II – DETERMINING THE AFFECTED CHANNEL

The therapist questions the dermis of the radial groove, at the distal level of the wrist.

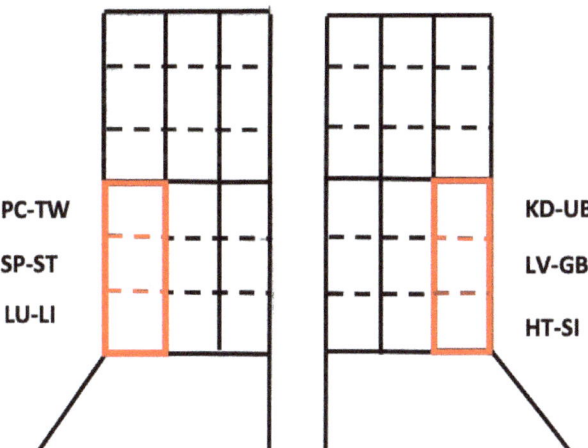

III – CORRECTION

The therapist sweeps across the channel(s) related to the blocked position on the wrist, along the pathway on the upper or lower limb (from the base of the limb to its extremity or in the other way), lightly stroking with his fingertips on the surface, until he feels a bump, an obstacle under his hand. He covers this zone 2 or 3 times until the blockage sensation disappears.

XXV – THE TENDINO-MUSCULAR CHANNELS (JING JIN)

The tendino-muscular (or sinew) channels are the most superficial ones. They begin at the extremity of the fingers and toes (Jing Well points), follow the course of the main channels on the surface and then converge in a zone of the upper body or head. They only convey the defensive energy (Wei Qi). An entry door for the external disturbing energies, they are also the first lines of defence against them before they penetrate the main channels. However, most of the stagnations in the sinew channels have an emotional origin, caused by fears, apprehensions, and mental tension. The organism may then produce too much Wei Qi; the danger is the counterflow of this excess Wei Qi which may burn up the organs in depth. The foot Yang sinew channels are the most frequently disturbed (mainly GB and ST; LI for the hand Yang ones).

I – PALPATORY STUDY

→ At the level of the toes and fingers:
The therapist takes the entire toe or the finger extremity between both hands that he brings closer with an "energetic" pressure and evaluates whether he can « cross » the bone or not.

impulse

Toe finger → no blockage

Toe finger → blockage

→ On the pathway of the tendino-muscular channel:
With one hand's outstretched fingertips, the therapist applies a vertical deep pres-

sure and evaluates whether he can" cross" the muscular layer or if he encounters a resistance, a barrier that keeps him from doing so.

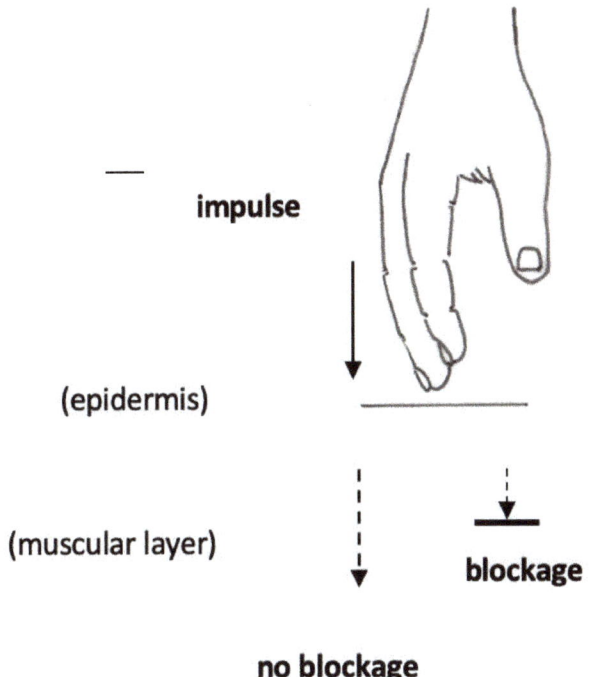

Reminder:

→ This palpation differs from the one of the main channels where the therapist, with his hand laid flat, lengthwise on their pathway, applies a vertical pressure on the surface and evaluates the epidermis response.

II – OVERALL CONTROL

→ Mid-lower border of the mandible body- the impulse is given in its axis- (dermis).
→ Distal half of the dorsal side of the 1st metacarpal bone (surface).

III – CORRECTION

The therapist grasps the toe or fingertip between his thumb and index finger. From this extremity on, the other hand gradually goes back up along the channel with a deep palpation of the muscular layer until he finds a rope.

After its loosening, the therapist controls whether the sinew channel is free through palpating the toe/ fingertip with both hands or the sinew channel on its pathway with one hand as described above. If it is not the case, he keeps going back up the channel until he finds a new rope and so on until its complete freeing.

Notes:

→ Stagnations in the tendino-muscular channels are often self-corrected in the course of treatment, that is why we do not start with a correction on this level. We control at the end of the session if there is still a blockage to remove.
→ In lumbar back pain, sciatica, the UB sinew channel is often disturbed.
→ **Case of the 3rd toe**: there is no point on the third toe, nor is there one on the vertebra T8. Both are in relation with the **Great Luo of the Stomach (Xu Li)**.

> Blockage confirmation through the surface palpation of the dorsal side of the index finger's third phalanx, below the nail.
> The correction is made with one hand grasping the third toe, the other hand, with a surface palpation, goes down along the Stomach channel on the lower limb until the therapist finds the rope. It releases tensions from the stomach to the left, the duodenum to the right and mostly from the diaphragm. This blockage is quite frequent.

XXVI – ELIMINATION FUNCTION OF ST 36 - ST 37 - ST 39 POINTS

It is the elimination function of these points at the level of the digestive tract that we study in this chapter:

- ST 36 ➡ the Lower He point of Stomach
- ST 37 ➡ the Lower He point of Large Intestine
- ST 39 ➡ the Lower He point of Small Intestine

I – OVERALL CONTROL

- ➔ Medial (inner) side of the 1st metatarsal base (dermis).
- ➔ Medial side of the knee, below the medial tuberosity of the tibia, at the SP 9-point level (surface).

The therapist looks for the closed point on the same side.

II – CORRECTION

- ➔ It is done with one hand on the closed point, the other looks for the rope on the related viscera.

XXVII – THE 3 DAN TIAN

Three major energetic centres called Dan Tian, a fundamental concept of the Daoist Tradition, are related to the three aspects of the Fire: Fire-Light (upper Dan Tian), Fire-Heat (lower Dan Tian) and both Light and Heat Fire (middle Dan Tian), and to the three forms of love as conceptualised by ancient Greek philosophy: Agape (upper Dan Tian), Philae (middle Dan Tian) and Eros (lower Dan Tian). They are seated on a very deep level. In practice, we find their disturbance in cases of mental illness, great anguishes or pathologies related to Yuan Qi (fire of Ming Men) which does not feed the lower Dan Tian any longer (internal cold, frigidity, impotence, infertility, pain and weakness in the lumbar region…).

The articulations of the thumb column are in resonance with the three Dan Tian:
- → The 1st metacarpal base is in resonance with the upper Dan Tian (located at the centre of the brain).
- → The 1st metacarpal head is in resonance with the middle Dan Tian (located in the Heart).
- → The interphalangeal articulation is in resonance with the lower Dan Tian (located in the lower burner).

I – OVERALL CONTROL

Through the surface interrogation of the middle finger's third phalanx, below the nail.

II – SPECIFIC CONTROL OF THE 3 DAN TIAN

It is done through an osseous vertical palpation of the thumb articulations. The therapist evaluates the response (the "elasticity", the rebound) of the bone.

III – CORRECTION

Two steps:
- → 1st step: the therapist with a light, vertical palpation "on the surface of the surface", looks for a zone which does not respond on the front midline of the body at the level of:
  - → Glabella (Yin Tang), for the upper Dan Tian.

XXVII – THE 3 DAN TIAN

- → Sternum, for the middle Dan Tian.
- → RM 4 zone, for the lower Dan Tian.

- → 2nd step: from this hand on the front side, the other one, still with a light palpation, looks for the rope on the back midline of the body, at the level of:
  - → Occipital area (DM 17 zone), for the upper Dan Tian.
  - → T4 – T5 – T6 zone, for the middle Dan Tian.
  - → DM 4 zone, for the lower Dan Tian.

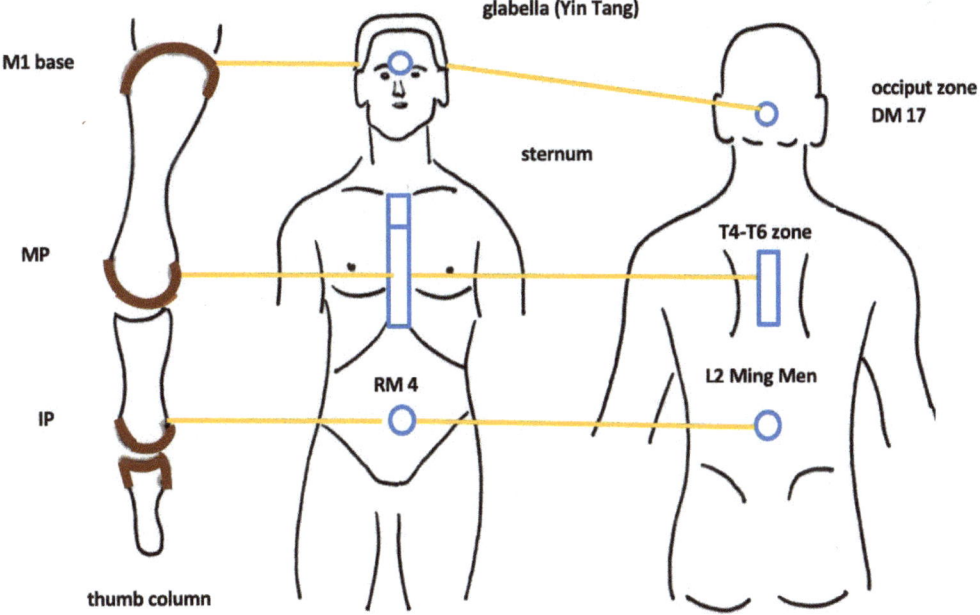

PLATE 35: THE 3 DAN TIAN

XXVIII – COMMENTS ON THE READING GRID

→ In all cases, after a complete treatment, the reading grid is "clean". All controls within the grid are blockage free, a sign that the organism has integrated all the given information.
The therapist may assess the efficiency of the initiated corrections, even in the course of the session, by going over the different controls studied in chapters II and III (hand decoding, muscle decoding, channel palpation, energy movement of the viscera), as well as the classic examination (pulse taking, abdomen palpation, etc.), and even the osteopathic examination (segmental mobility tests at the vertebral, peripheral, cranial and visceral levels). The points related to the disturbed energetic functions are open again, particularly, the 5 Shu points that the therapist may quickly review to make sure of it

→ It is determining to understand that the reading grid indicates only the blockages that need to be corrected, as the other ones are the consequence of the former. So, for example, not finding any blockage in the overall control of the Back-Shu/Front-Mu points does not mean that all the Back-Shu and Front-Mu points are open. If some are closed, the reason is to be found in other blockages in the reading grid. After the correction of the latter, these points are open again.

→ However, in chronic pathologies, the palpatory expression of the disease remains present. In a patient suffering from serious rheumatism, the Spleen channel on one side, the 1st metacarpal bone, the index finger's second phalanx, the tibialis posterior muscle, in resonance with the Spleen function, are not completely free. One of the 5 Shu points does not respond as clearly. The same holds true for the Kidney channel, the 3rd metacarpal bone in the case of chronic renal failure, or for the Triple Warmer channel in thyroid problems. In mental pathologies, the metacarpal blockages mainly appear through a surface palpation lengthwise and the disturbance is also found at the level of the small facial bones (see the hand decoding on plate 2). The treatment, then, enables the body to balance itself in the best possible way according to its abilities.

→ As it was mentioned above, all the blockages inside the reading grid are corrected. A precise order in the treatment is proposed, "from the densest to the most subtle":
  → At first, the elemental plane (channel circulation, master points, secondary Extraordinary Channels, general functions, Luo points, etc.) using the distal points of channels.
  → Then, the corporal plane (Back-Shu points, Front-Mu points, Ren Mai, Chong Mai, etc.)
  → Then, the emotional plane (emotional chains of Du Mai, Stomach, Gall Bladder

channels, the chain from KD 22 to KD 27…).
- → At last, the spiritual plane (Heart channel, the outer pathway of the UB channel, the 3 Dan Tian…).

→ The Energy (Qi) should not be only a vague concept but a tangible reality in hands. The "sensation" is what gives "sense" to our "action". Between our hands, an organ with a stagnation appears dense and heavy whereas it seems lightweight when the Energy flows in it freely. A "tight" skull, as if it were "caught in a vise", "breathes" again after treatment.

→ As described previously, when interrogating dermis areas horizontally with the fingers or the hand palm, the blockages which appear in all directions cannot be interpreted according to the reading grid. Note in that case that it is not possible to move the dermis on the underlying layer.

When interrogating epidermis areas horizontally with the fingers or the hand palm, the blockages which appear in all directions cannot be interpreted according the reading grid. In that case, the dermis right under the epidermis area can be mobilized on the underlying layer. The same goes for the osseous level.

Two aetiologies for these areas which blockages appear in all directions:
- → Either a structural problem: pathologies as, for instance, arthritis or arthrosis deformans, serious lymphoedema, adherent scar, etc., alter the structure of the tissue.
- → Or an energetic disorder:
  - → As for the dermis areas, the therapist will find mainly a disturbance in the Back-Shu points (Jing Bie or function), the Spleen chain or the traumatic centre and specially for the cranial dermis, in the tendino-muscular channels.
  - → As for the epidermis (surface) areas, the blockage will be in the emotional chains of Du Mai, Stomach and Gall Bladder channels.
  - → As for the osseous level, the therapist will find a disturbance in the Front-Mu points (Jing Bie or function).

After correction of the energetic disorder, the possible blockage appears in one direction.

→ It should be noted that the corrections made from the point/organ decoding proposed by J. PIALOUX, confirm the accuracy of his decoding

→ All palpatory subtleties have not been addressed in this book meant to be concise but the essence of our practice is largely described. We would like to draw attention to one last point: the vibratory environment of the therapist's office, the treatment room. The vibratory disturbances (electromagnetic, telluric, etheric, etc.) can induce "false" blockages which are not found in a "clean" environment. The influence of housing on health will be the subject of a forthcoming publication.

EPILOGUE

AND ANNEXES

EPILOGUE

Our approach to Chinese Medicine advances proposals which are based on the energetic palpation and a rigorous methodology. It reveals that the basic principles inherited from the Tradition are inscribed in the tissues of the human body. We encourage the reader to experiment on his own our working hypotheses and to overcome the initial palpating difficulties or the seeming complexity of the reading grid for it constitutes a reliable and effective tool in our practice as experience has shown us. However, this approach could not cover all aspects of the energetic system or be a substitute for certain classic techniques. Without a doubt, some new controls will come to complete or modify it, since, as for any science, we will never be done searching.

ANNEX I: SUMMARIZED PLATES

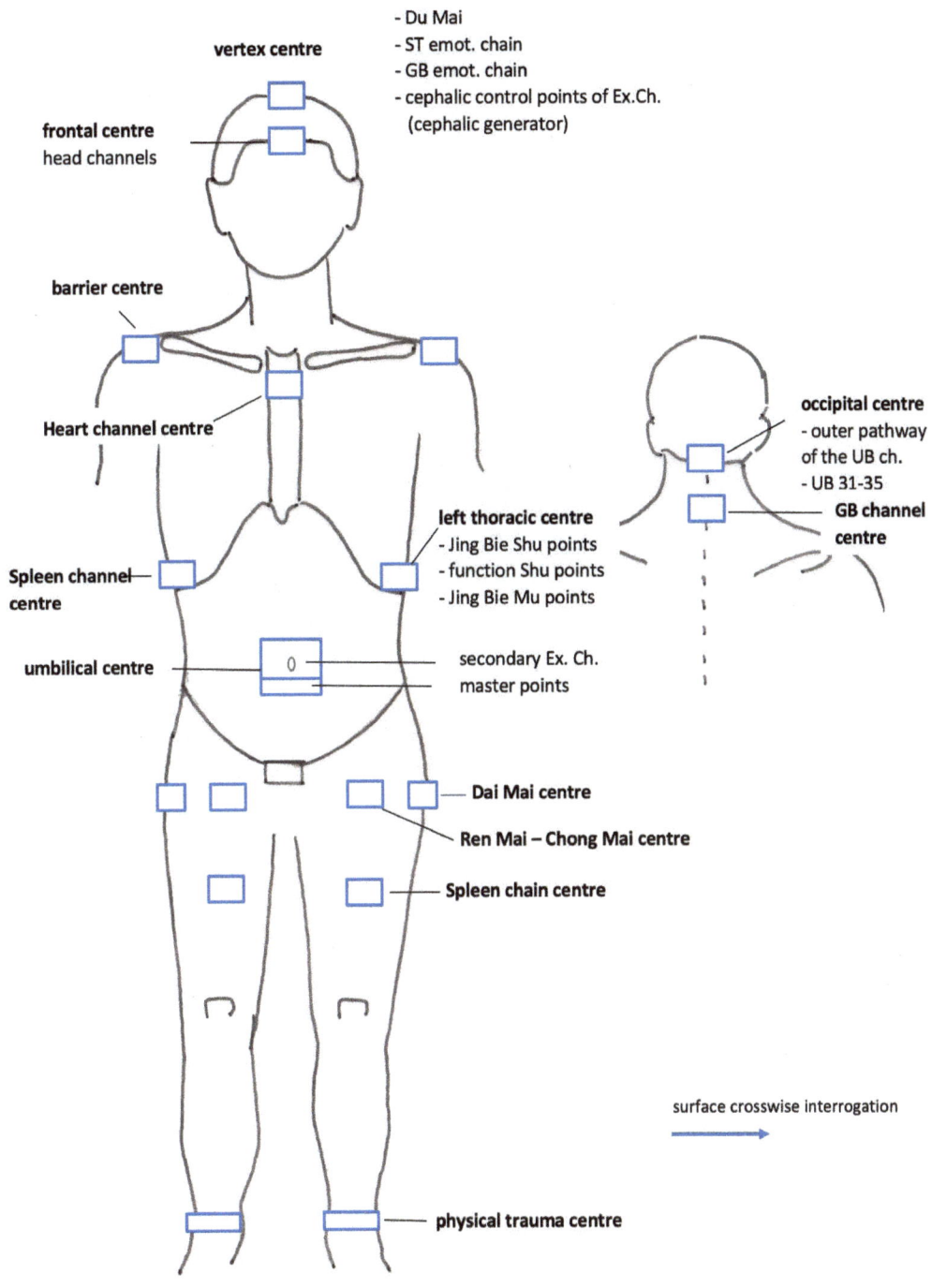

PLATE 36: THE CENTRES

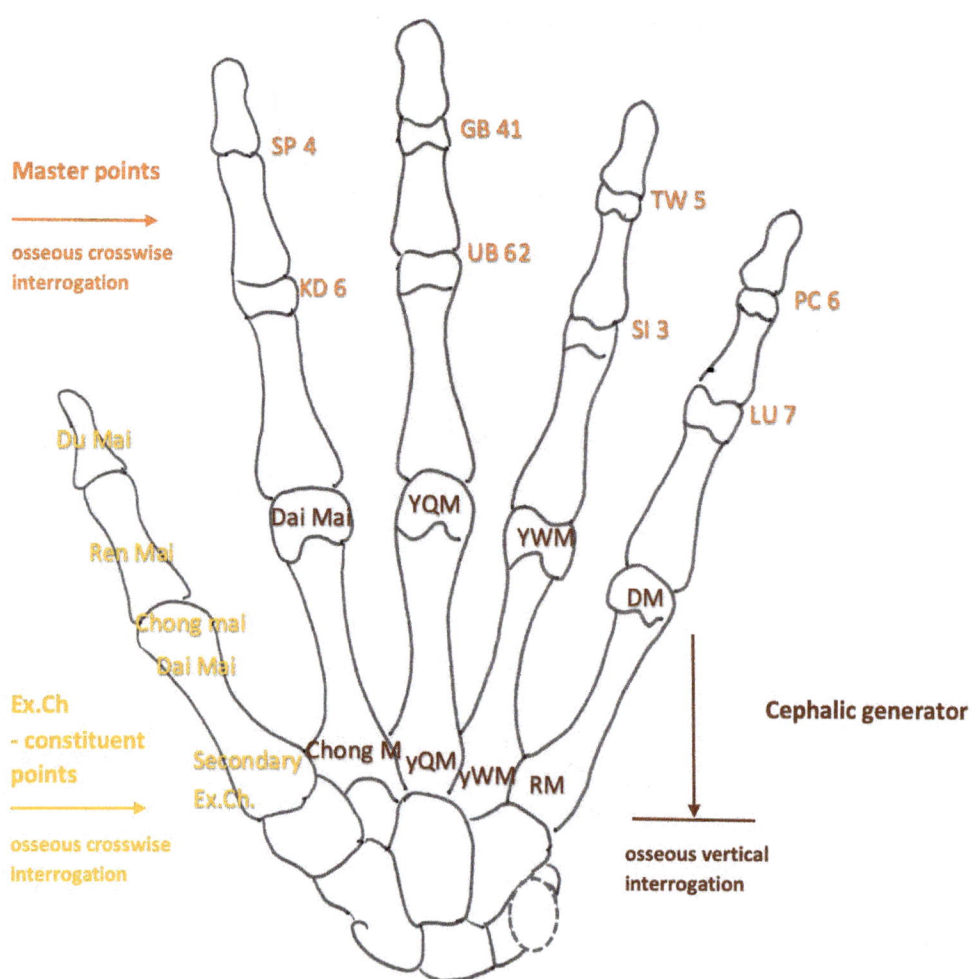

PLATE 37: THE EXTRAORDINARY CHANNELS ON THE HAND DORSAL SIDE (OSSEOUS)

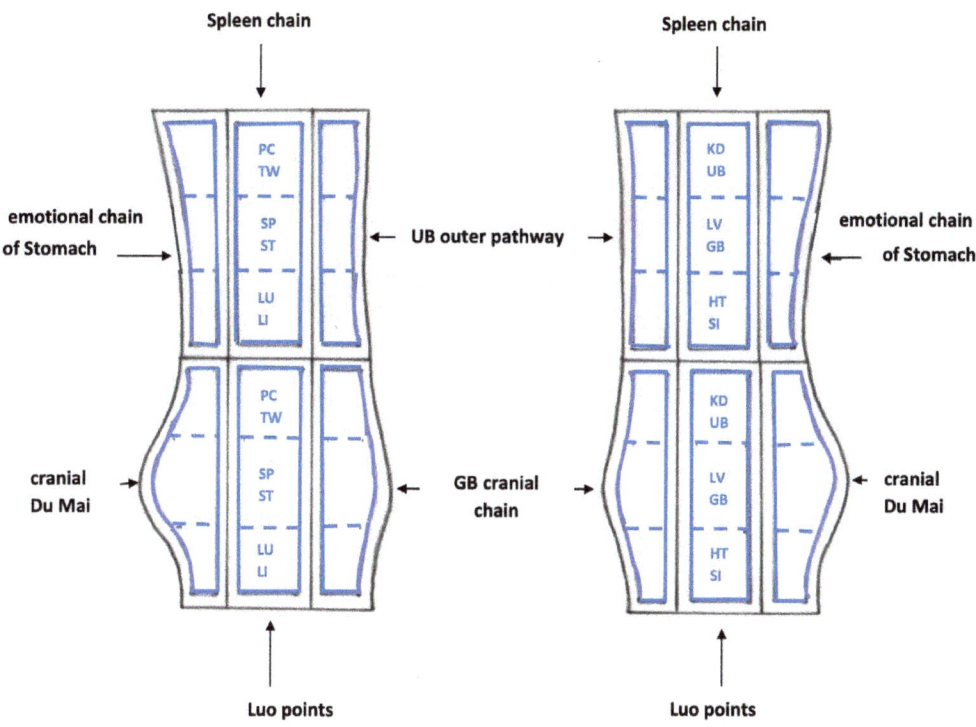

PLATE 38: THE ENERGETIC FUNCTIONS AT THE ANTERIOR SIDE OF THE WRIST (SURFACE)

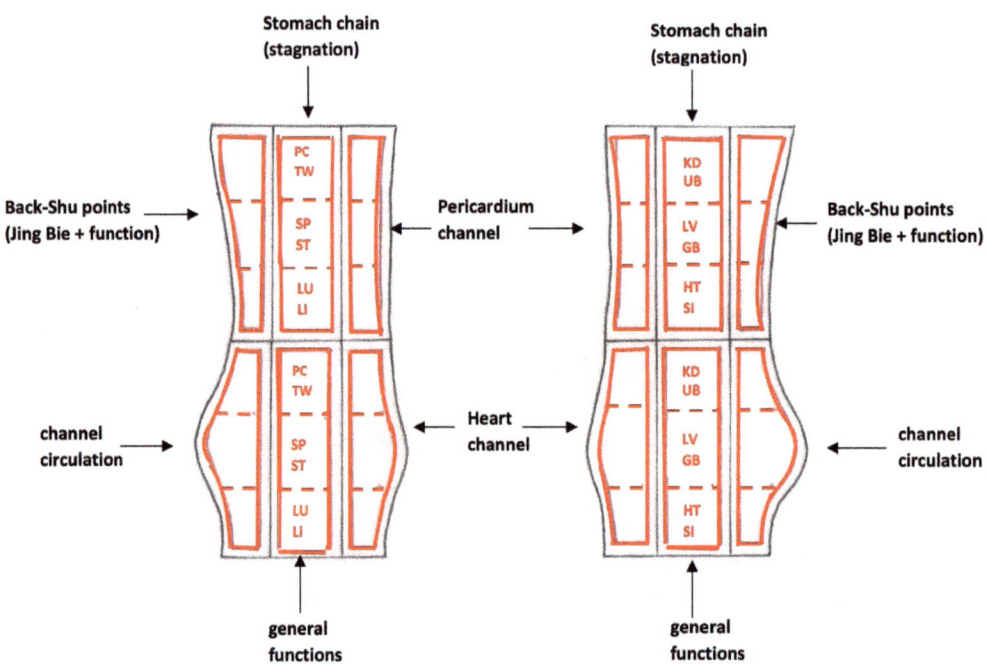

PLATE 39: THE ENERGETIC FUNCTIONS AT THE ANTERIOR SIDE OF THE WRIST (DERMIS)

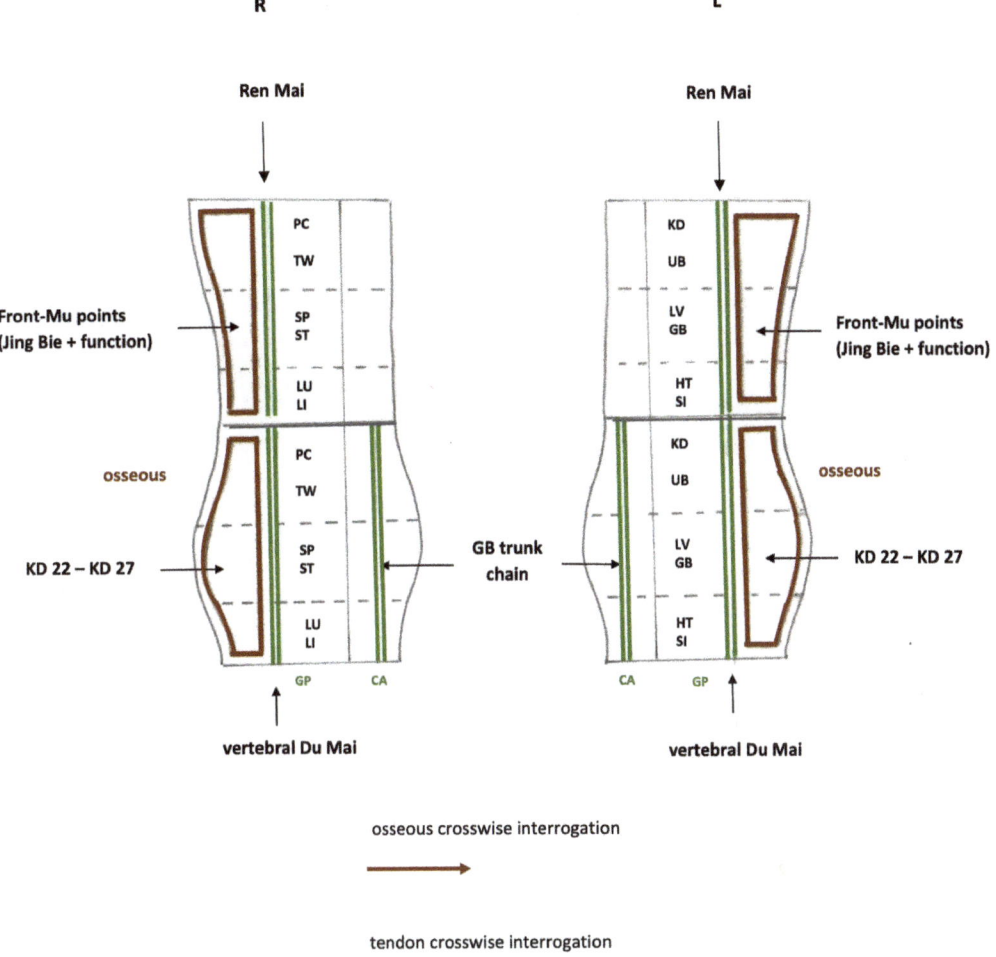

PLATE 40: THE ENERGETIC FUNCTIONS AT THE ANTERIOR SIDE OF THE WRIST (OSSEOUS + TENDON)

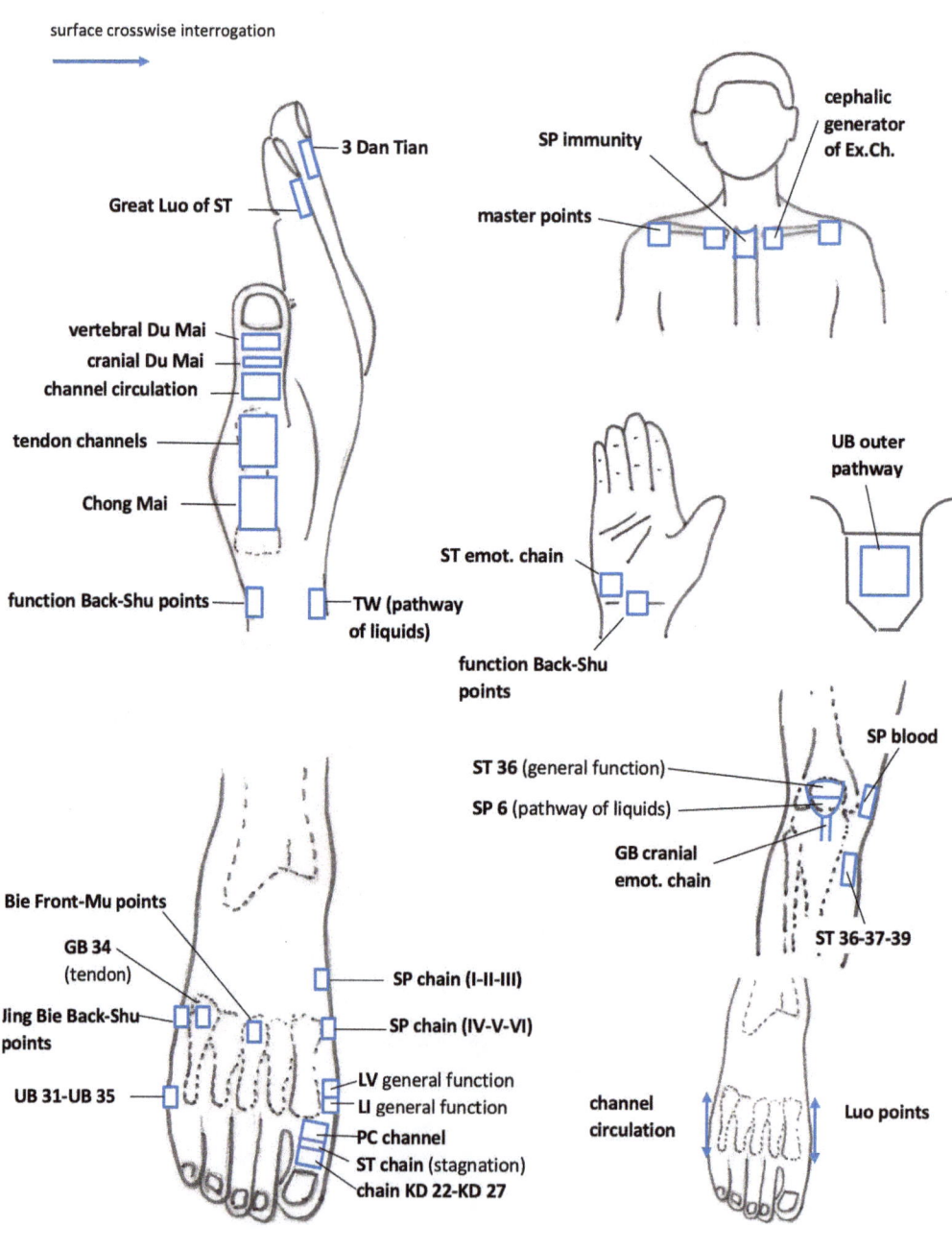

PLATE 41: SUMMARIZED PLATE (SURFACE)

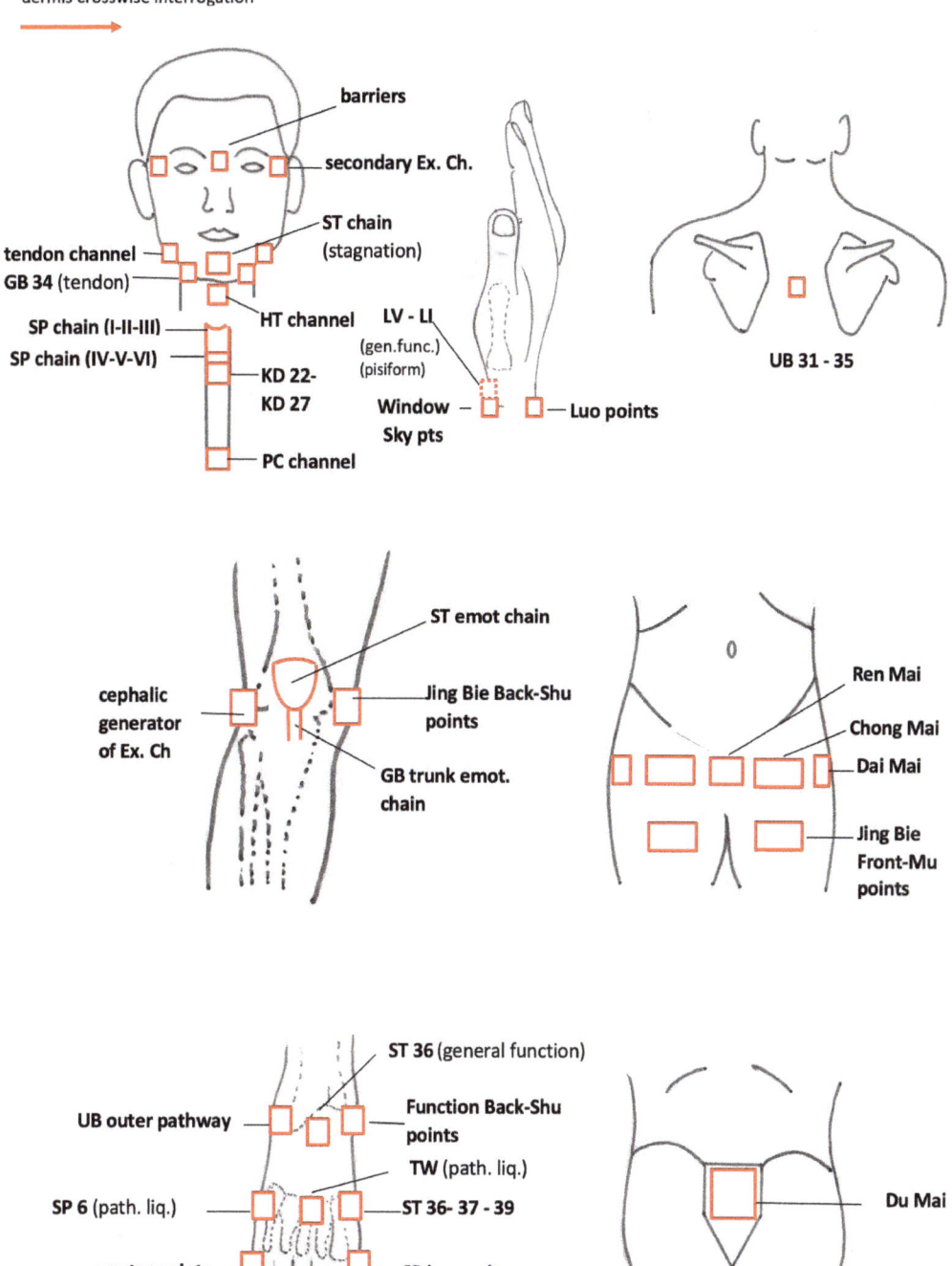

PLATE 42: SUMMARIZED PLATE (DERMIS)

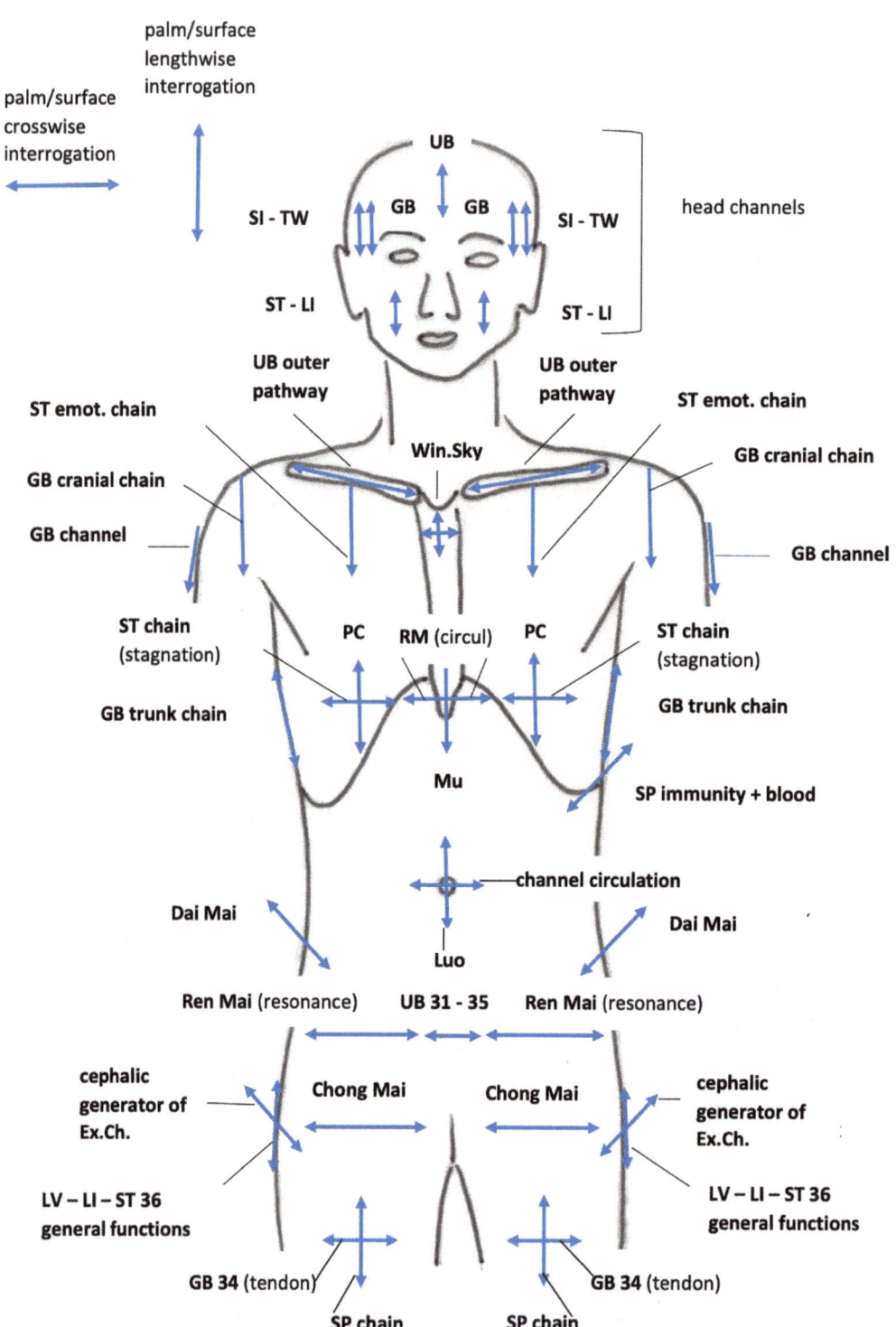

PLATE 43: SUMMARIZED PLATE (PALM/SURFACE) (I)

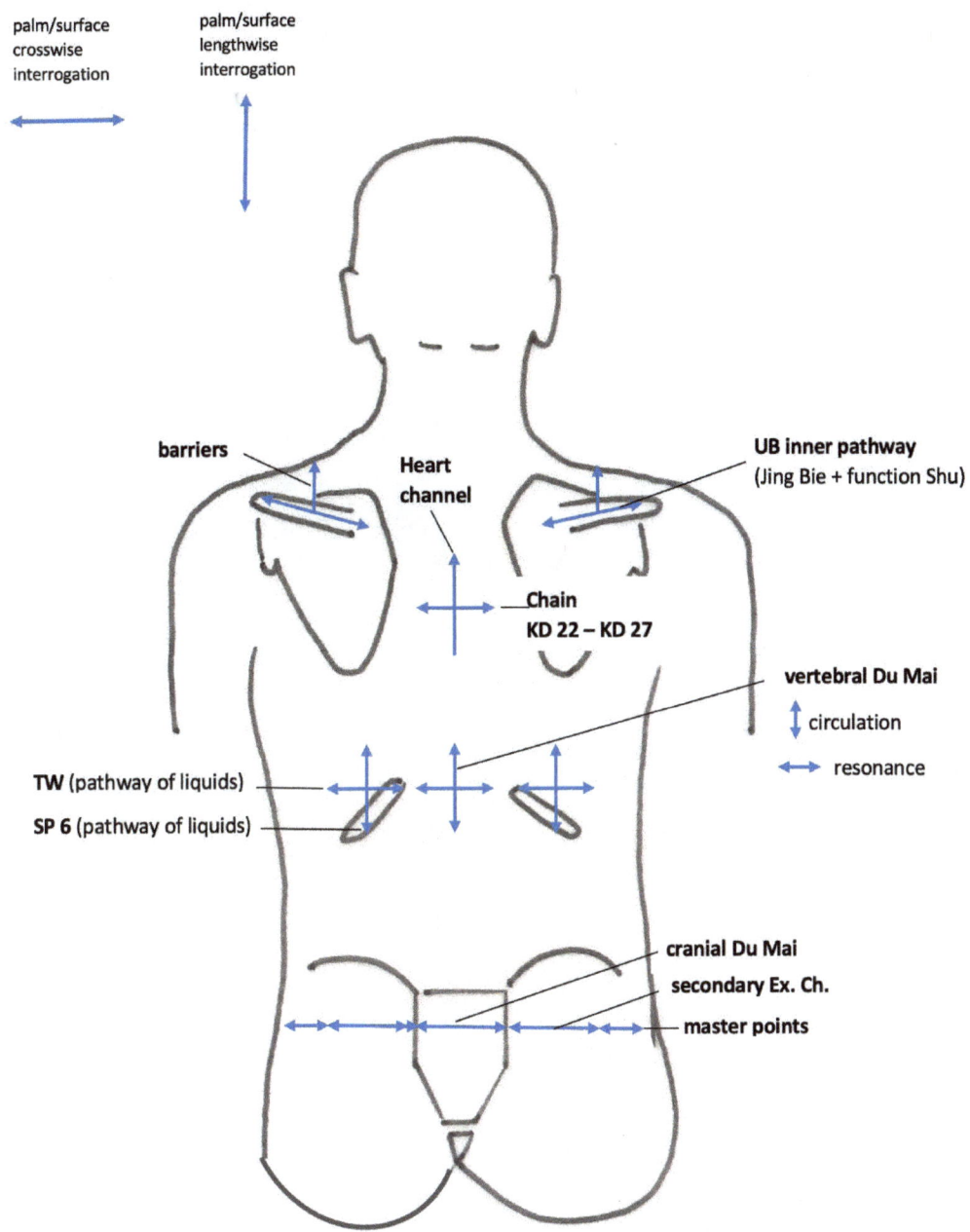

PLATE 44: SUMMARIZED PLATE (PALM/SURFACE) (II)

ANNEX II: BIBLIOGRAPHY

- Auteroche Bernard and Navailh Paul, *Le diagnostic en médecine chinoise*, Ed. Maloine
- Blin Régis, *L'hexagramme Tridimensionnel*, S.F.E.R.E
- Borsarello Jean, *Traité d'Acupuncture*, Ed. Masson
- Combe Yvon, *L'Homme Etoile*, Editions du Cosmogone
- Dürckheim Karlfried Graf, *Hara: The Vital Center of Man*, Inner Traditions Publisher
- Faubert André, "Traité Didactique d'Acupuncture Traditionnelle", Ed. Guy Trédaniel
- Focks Claudia, "Atlas d'Acupuncture", Ed. Elsevier Masson
- Grof Stanislav, "Realms of the Human Unconscious", Souvenir Press Ltd
- Grosjean Daniel and Benini Patrice, "Traité Pratique de Microkinésithérapie, vol. I-II-III-IV", CFM
- Guiliani Jean-Pierre, *L'Alphabet du Corps Humain*, Ed. Arkhana Vox.
- Maciocia Giovanni, *The Foundations of Chinese Medicine*, Churchill Livingstone Publisher
- Martin-Hartz Jacques and Pialoux Jacques, *Le Dragon de Jade*, Ed. Fondation Cornélius Celsus
- Pialoux Jacques, *Le Diamant Chauve Plus*, Ed. Fondation Cornélius Celsus
- Pialoux Jacques, *Guide to Acupuncture and Moxibustion*, Ed. Fondation Cornélius Celsus
- Schutzenberger Anne Ancelin, *The Ancestor syndrome: Transgenerational Psychotherapy and the Hidden Links in the Family Tree*, Routledge Publisher
- Senn Dominique, *La Balance Tropique*, Ed. Fondation Cornélius Celsus
- Souchard Philippe, *Rééducation Posturale Globale*, Ed. Elsevier Masson

ANNEX III: LIST OF ABBREVIATIONS

LU	→	Lung
LI	→	Large Intestine
ST	→	Stomach
SP	→	Spleen
HT	→	Heart
SI	→	Small Intestine
UB	→	Urinary Bladder
KD	→	Kidney
PC	→	Pericardium
TW	→	Triple Warmer
GB	→	Gall Bladder
LV	→	Liver
Ex.Ch.	→	Extraordinary Channel
RM	→	Ren Mai
DM	→	Du Mai
yQM	→	Yin Qiao Mai
YQM	→	Yang Qiao Mai
yWM	→	Yin Wei Mai
YWM	→	Yang Wei Mai

ACKNOWLEDGMENTS

I would like to thank all those who have shared with me their knowledge in the last thirty years.

In particular:

- Philippe Souchard, who has developed the "Rééducation Posturale Globale", in the spirit of Françoise Mezieres' method.
- Jacques Pialoux, Régis Blin and Jean-Pierre Guiliani, for their teachings and own vision of Traditional Chinese Medicine.
- Yvon Combe, for his synthesis between the Oriental medical and spiritual Traditions and the discoveries of the Occidental Energetic medicine, as Jacques Pialoux also did in several works.
- Daniel Grosjean and Patrice Benini, who have elaborated the "Microkinésithérapie", a manual therapy based on the energetic palpation, which utilizes its own reading grid of the body.

Thanks to all the yesterday's and today's great thinkers who, through their works, contributed to enrich my reflection. Among them and pell-mell:

Jean Charon, Régis Dutheil, Rupert Sheldrake, Trinh Xuan Thuan, Jean-Claude Ameisen, Matthieu Ricard, Karlfried Graf Dürckheim, Stanislas Grof, Carl Gustav Jung, Anne Ancelin Schutzenberger, David Tansley, Alice Bailey, Marcel Granet, Baruch Spinoza…

Thanks to Cyriane Jacques and Véronique Cherel for their careful reading of the manuscript and the layout of the book and to José Pirès for the beautiful front cover.

Thanks also to Michel Bosc and Julien Bringuier for their availability and patience in the English translation.

Denys Jacques

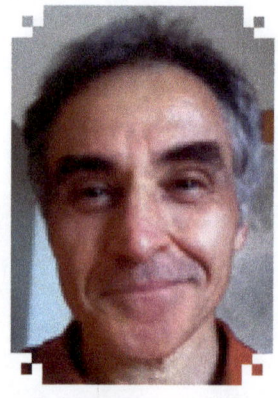

First, I would like to express my gratitude to my father, Denys Jacques who has transmitted his passion and the benefits of his experience gained over all these years of practice and research. For me, his teachings went beyond Chinese medicine.

Thanks also to Michael Smith, M.D. who was of great help in my personal development and, of course, to the members of the SFERE college, Yves Giarmon, Hervé De Coux, Jean-Pierre Guiliani and Régis Blin.

Thanks to Veronique Cherel.

Victor Jacques

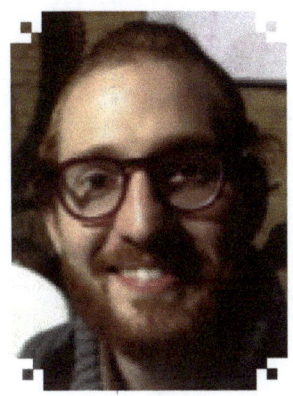

Discovery Publisher is a multimedia publisher whose mission is to inspire and support personal transformation, spiritual growth and awakening. We strive with every title to preserve the essential wisdom of the author, spiritual teacher, thinker, healer, and visionary artist.

www.ingramcontent.com/pod-product-compliance
Lightning Source LLC
Chambersburg PA
CBHW060923170426
43192CB00021B/2854